The Principles of Virtual Orthopedic Assessment

Khaled M. Emara · Nicolas S. Piuzzi
Editors

The Principles of Virtual Orthopedic Assessment

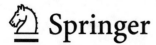
Springer

Editors
Khaled M. Emara
Department of Orthopedic Surgery
Ain Shams University
Cairo, Egypt

Nicolas S. Piuzzi
Department of Orthopedic Surgery
Cleveland Clinic Foundation
Cleveland, OH, USA

ISBN 978-3-030-80404-6   ISBN 978-3-030-80402-2   (eBook)
https://doi.org/10.1007/978-3-030-80402-2

This Springer imprint is published by the registered company Springer Nature Switzerland AG
The registered company address is: Gewerbestrasse 11, 6330 Cham, Switzerland

Foreword

Telemedicine has become an emerging necessity in the practice of orthopedic surgery following the paradigm shift brought on by the COVID-19 pandemic. The physical exam is a critical part of the orthopedic examination and also the most challenging to perform in a virtual encounter. Given the emerging importance of this skill and the relative paucity of literature on the methods for performing a virtual orthopedic exam, a group of interdisciplinary professionals came together in an attempt to address such knowledge gap and provide fellow providers as well as patients with tools to improve remote healthcare delivery. The work at hand is the combined effort of an international group of orthopedic surgeons from the Cleveland Clinic Foundation, Cleveland, Ohio and Ain Shams University, Cairo, Egypt. The Cleveland Clinic's Orthopedic Informatics Group has been a pioneer in developing workflows and its more recently developed model of musculoskeletal virtual triage currently provides remote urgent and emergent orthopedic care for over four million individuals in Northeast Ohio. Similarly, the Ain Shams University Group has been engaged in virtual musculoskeletal care, providing much needed tertiary support and referral services to much of the Middle East and North Africa. The conglomeration of both groups enabled the authors to identify areas of deficiency, conceptualize workflows, and provide recommendations on how to best conduct a virtual orthopedic examination regardless of the patient setting. We hope to contribute to the body of growing orthopedic literature on the topic and provide a comprehensive guide to our fellow practitioners as well as prospective patients.

Orthopedic Surgery   The Cleveland Clinic Orthopedic
Ain Shams University   Informatics Group
Cairo, Egypt

Preface

The use of technology for healthcare-related communication grew historically out of a need to treat patients located in remote areas who were physically distant from appropriate healthcare facilities and qualified medical professionals. Since then, telemedicine has expanded to myriad other applications, especially as a tool for providing convenient medical care to the modern, digitally connected, on-the-go patient. For these patients, telemedicine is not only convenient and compatible with their lifestyle, but it also reduces time wasted in waiting rooms and provides more direct access to physician care for minor but urgent conditions.

With the emergence of the global COVID-19 pandemic and the social distancing policies required to control the spread of infection, telemedicine has nearly entirely transformed from a convenient option to necessity across many specialties almost overnight. Unfortunately, orthopedic injury and disease continue to cause significant morbidity and mortality even as the pandemic rages on, and the need for orthopedic care remains.

Although telemedicine has a great capacity to augment the traditional face-to-face healthcare model with the tools of modern digital technology, there remain many components of the face-to-face encounter that are difficult to reproduce using telemedicine. One of the greatest difficulties of the telemedicine encounter is the clinical examination, for which many diagnostically vital steps cannot be assessed without face-to-face interactions. Although there are many elements that cannot be translated to a virtual setting, the ability to perform elements of this clinical examination virtually can provide a valuable option for evaluating and following up with orthopedic patients.

In this book, we will begin by briefly describing the history of telemedicine and different tools that may improve virtual orthopedic assessment. We will then outline the most state-of-the-art techniques and approaches for integrating medical history and possible telemedicine examination, broken down by body region. These virtual examination techniques are not meant to replace face-to-face consultations, which will still be required when a telemedicine visit fails to reach a definitive diagnosis, when cases are complex, and as a final check immediately prior to an invasive diagnostic or therapeutic procedure.

Cairo, Egypt   Khaled M. Emara
Cleveland, OH, USA   Nicolas S. Piuzzi

Contents

Editors and Contributors

About the Editors

Khaled M. Emara, MD, PhD, FEBOT, FRCS is the current Chairman of the SICOT bone infection committee and a Professor of Orthopedic Surgery at Ain Shams University of Cairo. Dr. Emara has been in practice for over 28 years and has trained as well as served a multitude of national and international communities. Dr. Emara joined the Faculty of Ain Shams University in 1994 after completing his residency at the same institution. He went on to do multiple trauma and pediatric orthopedic fellowships in Geneva; Switzerland, Toledo; Ohio, Dallas, Texas; and Portland, Oregon. Dr. Emara moved on to become the head of the education committee in the Egyptian Medical Syndicate, a position he held for 2 years (2011–2013) before dedicating his time to promoting orthopedic surgical education worldwide. In addition to being the Chairman of the SICOT's active infection committee, he is an engaged member of the trauma and fellowship committees, which offer surgeons high-quality surgical education worldwide and connects leaders in the field and potential mentors with aspiring orthopedic surgeons, forming life-long international bonds that persist beyond practice.

Dr. Emara is an avid researcher and a prolific author in some of the top Orthopedic Journals. He is also a fellow of the royal college of surgeons and a European Orthopedic Board-certified surgeon. In addition to teaching, Dr. Emara makes a point of engaging actively in humanitarian missions and care provision to in-need areas worldwide. He plans at least one relief mission annually and dedicates it to serve patients of various nationalities as well as those with diverse ethnic and religious backgrounds.

In addition to being a surgeon and a researcher, Dr. Emara is a loving husband and a father of three. His wife is an infectious disease physician and a Professor of microbiology.

Nicolas S. Piuzzi is an orthopedic surgeon specializing in adult joint reconstruction at Cleveland Clinic and currently serve as Adult Joint Reconstructive Surgery Research Director. As an orthopedic clinician-scientist, his expertise is in primary and revision total hip and knee procedures for the treatment of osteoarthritis, osteonecrosis, arthrofibrosis, osteolysis, periprosthetic infections, and periprosthetic fractures. As such, his research is directly translational to his clinical practice, reinforcing the clinician-scientist role. He is committed to the development and optimization of strategies for preservation, repair, regeneration, augmentation, or replacement of musculoskeletal tissues. Dr. Piuzzi vision is *to advance patient care through Evidence-Based Orthopedic Surgery and Personalized Medicine*.

As Staff Surgeon at Cleveland Clinic (CC) Adult Joint Reconstructive Surgery Center, he routinely performs 350+ surgeries per year. As Director of the Adult Joint Reconstruction Research Program, he was granted 40% dedicated time to coordinate and lead the CC Joints Clinical Research Program, a world leader team in arthroplasty research that incorporates translational and clinical research. As one of the largest and more productive Joints research groups in the United States, it has a total annual research expenditures exceeding $2 million from several funding sources and a staff team the comprises: one Program Manager, one Data Analyst, five Research Coordinators, and one Associate Staff (PhD), in addition to Research Fellows and Medical students. Altogether the group publishes 100+Peer-Reviewed manuscripts per year and is actively conducting 10+Clinical trials.

Along with his commitment to providing outstanding patient care and performing high quality impactful research, Dr. Piuzzi believes strongly in the importance of advancing the field of orthopedics through involvement in leadership, advocacy, and education, and is actively involved in mentoring medical students, residents, and fellows. He is a member of the American Academy of Orthopedic Surgeons (AAOS), Orthopedic Research Society (ORS), International Society for Cellular Therapy (ISCT), and American Association of Hip and Knee Surgeons (AAHKS) among others. He serves in the ORS Clinical Research Committee, AAOS American Joint Replacement Registry Young Committee, AAHKS Research Committee, and ISCT Musculoskeletal Committee. He has published over 220 peer-reviewed articles, presented in multiple national and international meetings, and won multiple awards including the 2018 AAOS/OREF/ORS Clinician Scholar Career Development Program Award and 2020 OREF/Current Concepts in Joint Replacement (CCJR) Clinical Practice Award. He currently serves as Associate Editor in the Journal of Knee Surgery and Journal of Hip Surgery, as well as reviewer in numerous prestigious Journals.

Contributors

Ramy Ahmed Diab Orthopedic Surgery, Ain Shams University, Cairo, Egypt

Keith Diamond Department of Orthopedic Surgery, Maimonides Medical Center, Brooklyn, NY, USA

Mahmoud Ahmed Elshobaky Orthopedic & Traumatology, Faculty of Medicine, Ain Shams University Hospital, Cairo, Egypt

Medicine/Surgery "MBBCh", Faculty of Medicine, Ain Shams University, Cairo, Egypt

Ahmed K. Emara Department of Orthopedic Surgery, Cleveland Clinic Foundation, Cleveland, OH, USA

Khaled M. Emara Department of Orthopedic Surgery, Ain Shams University, Cairo, Egypt

Michael Erossy Department of Orthopedic Surgery, Cleveland Clinic Foundation, Cleveland, OH, USA

Mohamed Noureldeen Essa Al Bank Al-Ahly Hospital, Cairo, Egypt

Peter Evans Department of Orthopedic Surgery, Cleveland Clinic Foundation, Cleveland, OH, USA

Mona Salah Mohamed Farhan Orthopedic & Traumatology, Faculty of Medicine, Ain Shams University Hospital, Cairo, Egypt

Healthcare & Hospital Management, American University in Cairo AUC, Cairo, Egypt

Orthopedic & Traumatology, General Air Force Hospital, Cairo, Egypt

Medicine/Surgery "MBBCh", Faculty of Medicine, Ain Shams University, Cairo, Egypt

Mostafa Gemeah Health Care Innovation Program, Arizona State University, Tempe, AZ, USA

Jason Genin Department of Orthopedic Surgery, Cleveland Clinic Foundation, Cleveland, OH, USA

Ahmed Abdel Salam Abdel Halim Orthopedic Surgery, Ain Shams University, Cairo, Egypt

Medicine and Surgery, Ain Shams University, Cairo, Egypt

Mohamed Amr Hemida Orthopedic Surgery, Ain Shams University, Cairo, Egypt

Carlos Higuera Department of Orthopedic Surgery, Cleveland Clinic Foundation, Cleveland, OH, USA

Dominic King Department of Orthopedic Surgery, Cleveland Clinic Foundation, Cleveland, OH, USA

Viktor Krebs Department of Orthopedic Surgery, Cleveland Clinic Foundation, Cleveland, OH, USA

Shady Abdelghaffar Mahmoud Orthopedic Surgery, Ain Shams University, Cairo, Egypt

Sara Lyn Miniaci-Coxhead Department of Orthopedic Surgery, Cleveland Clinic Foundation, Cleveland, OH, USA

Thomas Mroz Department of Orthopedic Surgery, Cleveland Clinic Foundation, Cleveland, OH, USA

Mitchell Ng Department of Orthopedic Surgery, Maimonides Medical Center, Brooklyn, NY, USA

Stephen Pinney Department of Orthopedic Surgery, Cleveland Clinic Foundation, Cleveland, OH, USA

Nicolas S. Piuzzi Department of Orthopedic Surgery, Cleveland Clinic Foundation, Cleveland, OH, USA

Jonathan Schaffer Department of Orthopedic Surgery, Cleveland Clinic Foundation, Cleveland, OH, USA

Joseph Styron Department of Orthopedic Surgery, Cleveland Clinic Foundation, Cleveland, OH, USA

Kevin Zhai Department of Orthopedic Surgery, Cleveland Clinic Foundation, Cleveland, OH, USA

Introduction

1

Khaled M. Emara, Shady Abdelghaffar Mahmoud,
and Nicolas S. Piuzzi

In the vast world of healthcare, applications of telemedicine are not only limited to direct patient care and can also include laboratory and radiological assessment, education and training, research, administration, and other meetings. Modalities of telemedicine also abound, and include telephone communication, video conferences, live text-based chat, asynchronous consultations using email or other store-and-forward applications, and remote patient monitoring using connected devices [1–3].

With the emergence of the global COVID-19 pandemic and the social distancing policies required to control the spread of infection, telemedicine has nearly entirely transformed from a convenient option to necessity across many specialties almost overnight. Unfortunately, orthopedic injury and disease continue to cause significant morbidity and mortality even as the pandemic rages on, and the need for orthopedic care remains. In the midst of such a pandemic, telemedicine provides an exceptional set of tools for physicians to continue diagnosing, treating, and managing orthopedic conditions.

The recent substantial growth in the field of digital health facilitates the rise of telemedicine. With a wide variety of mobile health apps and mobile medical devices, patients are starting to monitor and track their own health. These tools enable patients to diagnose their own infections, monitor glucose levels, and measure blood pressure using simple medical devices in their own homes. These consumer digital health devices can thus reduce the need for patients to see their doctors face-to-face. Telemedicine also confers many other benefits to patients and physicians alike:

K. M. Emara (✉)
Department of Orthopedic Surgery, Ain Shams University, Cairo, Egypt

S. A. Mahmoud
Orthopedic Surgery, Ain Shams University, Cairo, Egypt

N. S. Piuzzi
Department of Orthopedic Surgery, Cleveland Clinic Foundation, Cleveland, OH, USA
e-mail: piuzzin@ccf.org

greater access to physicians across the boundaries of space and time, increased patient comfort, increased data transmission security, lower costs. In addition, the increasing digitization of healthcare driven by telemedicine can fortify medical databases that may also offer benefits to potential research and quality improvement efforts [4, 5].

Although telemedicine has a great capacity to augment the traditional face-to-face healthcare model with the tools of modern digital technology, there remain many components of the face-to-face encounter that are difficult to reproduce using telemedicine. One of the greatest difficulties of the telemedicine encounter is the clinical examination, for which many diagnostically vital steps cannot be assessed without face-to-face interactions [1].

The orthopedic clinical examination is an essential factor in reaching an accurate diagnosis and providing the best management options. Although there are many elements that cannot be translated to a virtual setting, the ability to perform elements of this clinical examination virtually can provide a valuable option for evaluating and following up with orthopedic patients [6, 7]. In this book, we will begin by briefly describing the history of telemedicine and different tools that may improve virtual orthopedic assessment. We will then outline the most state-of-the-art techniques and approaches for integrating medical history and possible telemedicine examination, broken down by body region. These virtual examination techniques are not meant to replace face-to-face consultations, which will still be required when a telemedicine visit fails to reach a definitive diagnosis, when cases are complex, and as a final check immediately prior to an invasive diagnostic or therapeutic procedure. Nonetheless, the methods outlined in this book may provide a valuable addition to an orthopedic surgeon's arsenal when caring for a patient virtually.

References

1. Matusitz J, Breen GM. Telemedicine: its effects on health communication. Health Commun. 2007;21(1):73–83.
2. Wootton R, Craig J, Patterson V. Introduction to telemedicine. Boca Raton: CRC Press; 2017.
3. Conrad K. Making telehealth a viable component of our national health care system. Prof Psychol Res Pract. 1998;29(6):525.
4. Breen GM, Matusitz J. An evolutionary examination of telemedicine: a health and computer-mediated communication perspective. Soc Work Public Health. 2010;25(1):59–71.
5. Tuner JW, Thomas R, Reinsch NL. Willingness to try a new communication technology. J Bus Commun. 2004;41(1):5–26.
6. Daruwalla ZJ, Wong KL, Thambiah J. The application of telemedicine in orthopedic surgery in Singapore: a pilot study on a secure, mobile telehealth application and messaging platform. JMIR Mhealth Uhealth. 2014;2(2):e28.
7. Prada C, Izquierdo N, Traipe R, Figueroa C. Results of a new telemedicine strategy in traumatology and orthopedics. Telemed e-Health. 2020;26(5):665–70.

Infrastructure and Process

2

Ramy Ahmed Diab, Ahmed Abdel Salam Abdel Halim,
and Mohamed Amr Hemida

2.1 Purposes and Mechanism of Delivery

Telemedicine can be used for a variety of purposes, although this book focuses on the application of telemedicine to **direct patient care**. This includes the use of audio, video, and medical data between a patient and physician in establishing a diagnosis and treatment plan. Telemedicine can also be used by a general practitioner in consulting a specialist for **specialist referral services** in the diagnosis and/or treatment of a disease. Patients can also use devices such as a wearable electrocardiogram (ECG) monitor or serum glucose monitor to collect and send data to a **patient monitoring** center. Outside of patient care, telemedicine can also be used to provide **medical education** for both students and health professionals, an application whose demand dramatically increased with the COVID-19 pandemic [1, 2].

In the case of patient care, the **mechanism of telemedicine delivery** can also vary. **Closed network programs** link tertiary care hospitals with their outpatient clinics and health centers in rural or suburban areas with high-speed lines for telecommunication links between sites. There are 200 telemedicine networks in the United States using these programs. **Point-to-point connections** apply a similar principle as the closed network programs, linking hospitals with private networks to independent medical service providers at ambulatory care sites. Telemedicine can also be delivered more directly to patients through **health provider to home connections**, in which healthcare providers connect directly with patients over phone or teleconferencing systems for interactive clinical consultations. This same concept

R. A. Diab (✉) · M. A. Hemida
Orthopedic Surgery, Ain Shams University, Cairo, Egypt

Ahmed Abdel Salam Abdel Halim
Orthopedic Surgery, Ain Shams University, Cairo, Egypt

Medicine and Surgery, Ain Shams University, Cairo, Egypt

can be expanded to include consultations with home health nurses, nursing homes, and assisted living facilities. Physicians can also directly monitor patients using a **direct patient to monitoring center** mechanism. Remote monitoring of devices such as pacemakers allows the patients to preserve independent lifestyles. Finally, **web-based e-health patient service sites** can provide direct services over the internet [2].

2.2   Infrastructure

Hardware. Telemedicine can be conducted using a variety of different physical **devices**: desktop computer, laptop computer, cell phone (iOS or Android), or tablets. Windows 98 or an equivalent are the minimum operating system requirements. Most applications will run even on low-function devices, and the specific device suitability can and should be evaluated during a technical support pre-visit. Most of these devices have built-in **camera** and **microphone** suitable for telemedicine. However, desktop computers may not have these built-in, and an external webcam or microphone may be required. Options for these devices abound and are available at a low price [3, 4].

Network Connection. Most devices can connect to the network through **wireless** or **cable internet**. To ensure adequate quality and stability for a video encounter, download speed should be at least 15 Mbps and upload speed should be at least 5 Mbps. A **cellular network** such as 4G can be suitable for smartphone users and may provide an alternative option for computer users in the case of an unstable wireless internet connection if the cellular signal in the area is strong [3–5].

Video Platform. There are many video platforms that can be used in video conference consultations. Commonly used consumer video platforms such as Skype, Zoom, Google Duo, etc. can be very accessible. Other common platforms such as Cisco WebEx can provide greater encryption and additional security, although they may not be as familiar to the average user [3, 4].

Software. The introduction of technology has greatly impacted medicine, and numerous applications and software have been developed that now play a valuable role in medical assessment. In the orthopedic setting, **gait analysis software** can improve the quality of assessment by using computerized motion analysis to assess gait deviations. For example, Cortex by Motion Analysis is a fully integrated motion capture analysis software package that captures, processes, measures, and reports movement data. Hudl Technique Slow Motion Video Analysis by Ubersense Inc. is another example that analyzes motion using slow motion videos. Virtual **goniometer** applications provide easy and accurate ROM readings whether passive or active. They are useful for both initial consultations and follow-up visits to assess treatment efficacy [3, 4]. Virtual goniometers can also be used for X-ray measurements. In the table below is a list of goniometer applications and their developers: (Table 2.1).

Table 2.1 Goniometer applications

Program	Version	Developer
PT Goniometer	Version 1.2	Mark Busman
yROM Goniometer	Version 1.7.1	David Zhu
Goniometer Pro	Version 2.7	5fuf5
Goniometer	Version 1.2	June Gaming
Freeform Hip Goniometer	Version 1.2.1	Hip ROM, simplified
DrGoniometer	Version 2.3	CDM S.r.L
DynamicGoniometerAR	Version 1.5	Nikolaos Papadimitriou
Orthophical	Version 1.3	Alaa Al Adnani
ARorthopaedicGoniometer	Version 3.0	Nikolaos Papadimitriou
Goniometer	Version 1.1	Omari Saporta
ROM	Version 1.0.21	Range of monitor
Smart Goniometer	Current version 1.1.4	Smartex s.r.l
Goniometer Records	Version 1.03	Indian Orthopedic Research Group
Angulus	Version 3.1.5	DPP
Angles Video Goniometer	Version 1.2.1	Nathaniel Cochrane

The Physician's Room. The **lighting** should be adjusted to avoid extra brightness or darkness that could impact visibility. The conference itself should take place in a **private** room with a locked door, whether the visit is conducted from the physician's home, clinic, or a tertiary center. No other health worker should be in the room without the patient's knowledge and consent. To maximize **sound** quality and minimize distractions to the patient, mobile phone notifications should be silenced and any other kind of machine that might make sounds like printers should be turned off or disabled. If possible, the room should be soundproofed. The **camera** should be positioned at eye level in front of the physician to allow for proper communication [6].

2.3   Process for the Physician

Video Conference Etiquette. Appropriate **training** from technical support staff is required for a successful implementation of the telemedicine service and to ensure the physician's ability to deal with technology and the patient with harmony. Before beginning the telemedicine encounter, the physician should test the equipment, organize the background, lock the door, silence cell phones, and turn off any other sources of noise or distraction. Professional **attire** is important, and striped shirts, dark colors, or anything too visually distracting should be avoided. Maintaining **eye contact** with the patient throughout the encounter is essential for establishing rapport, and the camera should be placed in position to allow for that. As in the face-to-face encounter, it is important for the physician to **introduce themselves** at the beginning of the encounter, and to introduce any others who join the video conference. Especially in the virtual setting, it is important to **speak clearly** and articulate sounds carefully, as there are many potential technical barriers that impede sound transmission. If the patient is unable to hear, the physician should check the microphone volume and connection and **should not shout or yell** in an attempt to be heard. The physician should avoid monotonous speech and check the patient's understanding regularly using the teach-back method. Ultimately, **patience** will be key especially with potential technical barriers in communication. The patient should be given time to speak comfortably, and the physician should wait for 3 s after the patient has completed a thought to avoid possible interruption. Any unnecessary **body movement** by the physician should be kept to a minimum to avoid distracting the patient. Finally, a **smile** can go a long way to build rapport and develop the physician's relationship with the patient [6, 7].

Before the Telemedicine Visit. It is generally best to have technical support staff contact the patient prior to the visit and pre-test the video conference set-up to ensure everything is ready and troubleshoot any technical difficulties. The technical support team can also verify the physician's technical set-up and ensure that imaging studies are ready if available. A checklist of required equipment and instructions can be sent to both the physician and patient to ensure everything is in order. It is important to have backup contact information for patients to get in touch if any problems arise during the encounter. The technical support team can also coordinate the scheduling system for virtual visits, ensure delivery of any illustrations prepared by the physician, and assist patients with uploading any laboratory or imaging studies to the video conference platform [6, 7].

During the Telemedicine Visit. The physician should ensure that the patient understands the conversation using the teach-back methods and answer any questions that the patient may have. If any specific motions or maneuvers are required from the patient, supplementary documentation such as images or videos can be used as an adjunct [6].

After the Telemedicine Visit. As in any face-to-face encounter, the physician should **document** any findings, the duration of the visit, and any recordings or images captured during the consultation. The telemedicine coordinator can then send the patient a survey to rate the service and follow-up with them in order to improve the service [6, 7].

2.4   Process for the Patient

Before the Telemedicine Visit. At the time the visit is scheduled, a **consent** form should be provided for the patients to complete and return to the caregivers prior to the appointment. The telemedicine coordinator can help walk the patient through the consent process, should assistance be required. Once the appointment has been scheduled, patients should be sent a **checklist** for the region that needs to be assessed. The checklist should contain illustrations of any specific movements or maneuvers they will need to perform for the exam, and equipment or tools they will need to prepare before the visit, and details for how to configure their camera, furniture, lighting, and the general space from which they will join the video conference. Supplementary videos and images may be helpful to provide at this juncture as well. The patient should then be encouraged to **upload** any relevant laboratory, radiographic, or conduction studies prior to the visit, so that the service provider can integrate the studies into the virtual assessment and ensure that the provider. This data can provide important diagnostic value and improve accuracy for virtually triaging patients that will need to proceed to a full face-to-face appointment prior to definitive diagnosis. It is important to establish **billing** procedures as well for any charges associated with the visit, and ensure any technical complications are resolved. Options for digital payments include PayPal, Google Wallet, Apple Payment, and many others. Mobile wallets are another option that is accessible and feasible [6].

The following table (Table 2.2) can be shared with the patient in order to prepare them for the visit. It can put the patient at ease by letting them know what to expect and help them prepare for a comfortable and productive visit [6, 8].

Table 2.2 Patient's preparation for the visit checklist

General information about your upcoming virtual visit
Prior to your virtual visit
Read and complete the consent form in its entirety.
Upload all relevant imaging studies, conduction studies, and laboratory investigations to the system to be reviewed by the physician prior to the virtual assessment.
Read the checklist completely and prepare the necessary tools and settings before the assessment.
Test camera and headphone suitability to the video conferencing software. [A link should be provided for this test.]
During your virtual visit
Your visit will be divided into three components. First, your physician will take a **history** by conducting a face-to-face interview with you to ask you about any symptoms and complaints. The physician will ask you several questions to further analyze these symptoms, and may ask you about any other relevant details, past medical history, and family history. All of these questions will be targeted, concise, and focused on the region of concern. Second, your physician will perform a **clinical examination** and will ask you to expose the region of your body that is the subject of the visit. Usually, the examination involves looking at the region, observing your gait if needed, asking for your help to identify the exact region of pain, moving the examined joints, and potentially some special maneuvers that may help the physician reach a diagnosis. Finally, the physician will make a **recommendation** based on the medical information you uploaded and the exam. Your physician will recommend further investigations, indicate a need for face-to-face assessment, or make a definitive diagnosis and initiate a treatment plan.

(continued)

Table 2.2 (continued)

General information about your upcoming virtual visit

Important settings

Camera. The camera should be stabilized on a flat surface if not built-in to the computer and should be at the following levels. For an **upper extremity** exam (shoulder, elbow, hand) or a **spine** exam, the camera should be 4–5 ft (1.2–1.5 m) above the ground (Fig. 2.1). For a **lower extremity** exam (hip, knee, foot), the camera should be 2–3 ft (0.6–0.9 m) above the ground (Fig. 2.2a, b). For a **pediatric** exam, the camera should be adjusted based on the child's height and can generally be adjusted 2 ft (0.6 m) lower relative to the adult's adjustment. For **distance**, the camera should be kept 8 ft (1.8 m) away.

Light. Adequate light will help your physician provide a better inspection and a more accurate assessment. Avoid placing the camera in front of windows, as this may produce a harsh glare. Instead, keep the curtains closed and choose a quiet background to avoid physician distraction.

Furniture. Prepare the following for effective assessment, based on the region being examined.

- Spine: couch, chair.
- Shoulder: chair.
- Elbow: chair.
- Hand: desk.
- Hip: couch, chair.
- Knee: couch, chair.
- Foot and Ankle: couch, chair.

Room. Select a room that is convenient for such assessment, ideally already containing the requisite pieces of furniture. Choosing a closed space is generally preferred not only to protect your confidentiality but also to improve sound insulation and enable better communication with your physician. Ensure that there is adequate floor space (3 m × 1.5 m) to allow your physician to observe your walk.

Clothing. It is important to choose appropriate clothing so that your physician can adequately examine you. To ensure adequate exposure, please wear the following for your visit, depending on the region you want your physician to examine.

- Spine: underwear only.
- Shoulder: no shirt, pants only.
- Elbow: no shirt, pants only.
- Hand: exposed arms at least to the shoulders.
- Hip: underwear only.
- Knee: underwear only.
- Foot and Ankle: exposed legs at least to above the knees, bare feet.

Diagnostic tools

Please prepare the following items prior to the assessment, based on the region your physician will be assessing:

- Spine: cotton and black marker.
- Shoulder: cotton, bag, and black marker.
- Elbow: cotton and black marker.
- Hand: cotton, pen, key, bag, paper, and black marker (Fig. 2.3).
- Hip: cotton and black marker.
- Knee: cotton, pen, and black marker.
- Foot and Ankle: cotton and black marker.

Supplementary Images and Videos

Whether you are the patient or the assisting caregiver, we recommend that you view the supplementary images and videos to help conduct certain tests.

Fig. 2.1 Photo determines the distance and level of camera during the assessment of upper limb regions (shoulder, elbow, and hand) and spine

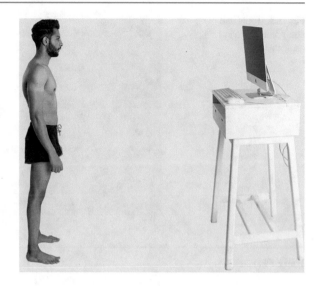

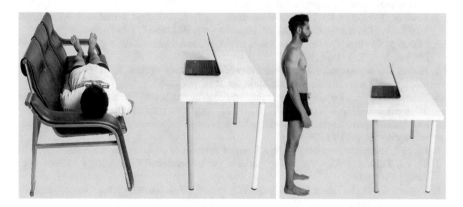

Fig. 2.2 (**a**, **b**) Photos determine the distance and level of camera during the assessment of lower limb regions (hip, knee, and foot) and pediatrics

Fig. 2.3 Tools and equipment for hand assessment

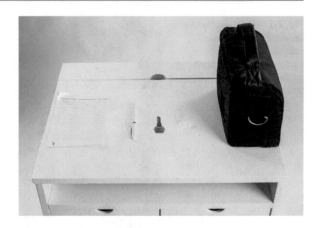

References

1. Darkins AW, Cary MA. Telemedicine and telehealth: principles, policies, performance, and pitfalls. New York: Springer; 2000. p. 218–20.
2. Zanaboni P, Wootton R. Adoption of telemedicine: from pilot stage to routine delivery. BMC Med Inform Decis Mak. 2012;12(1):4. https://doi.org/10.1186/1472-6947-12-1.
3. Maheu M, Whitten P, Allen A. E-health, telehealth, and telemedicine: a guide to startup and success. New York: Wiley; 2002.
4. Kornak J. System requirements for delivery of telemedicine services. In: Telemanagement of inflammatory bowel disease. Cham: Springer; 2016. p. 117–51.
5. Practice guidelines for videoconferencing-based telemental health. Washington, DC: American Telemedicine Association; 2009. p. 18–27. http://www.americantelemed.org/resources/telemedicine-practice-guidelines/telemedicine-practice-guidelines/videoconferencing-based-telemental-health#.VRGB8vnF9g0.
6. Major J. Telemedicine room design. J Telemed Telecare. 2005;11(1):10.
7. Shih J, Portnoy J. Tips for seeing patients via telemedicine. Curr Allergy Asthma Rep. 2018;18(10):50.
8. Viegas SF, Dunn K. Telemedicine—practicing in the information age. Philadelphia: Lippincott-Raven Publishers; 1998. p. 316–7.

Shoulder and Upper Arm

3

Mohamed Amr Hemida, Kevin Zhai, Dominic King,
and Jason Genin

3.1   Overview

Shoulder problems are a common complaint with orthopedic patients, and examination can be readily translated to a virtual setting. Virtual orthopedic assessment of different shoulder pathologies can have a significant impact on patient outcomes and satisfaction by reaching an accurate diagnosis and offering appropriate management options, whether conservative or surgical treatment.

There are three components of the virtual orthopedic shoulder examination. The first component is history taking, which has an especially high impact in the virtual setting and serves to provide a foundation and roadmap for the entire visit. Examination is the next component, which requires the most adjustment from the in-person to the virtual setting. Finally, by combining the results of these first two components, the physician can order the required studies (laboratory or radiological) to reach the final diagnosis [1, 2].

One of the most common shoulder pathologies involves the rotator cuff tendon (and the subacromial bursa), which may become compressed underneath the acromion during glenohumeral movement and give rise to pain and disturbance of the scapulothoracic rhythm. The most common site of impingement is subacromial, causing a painful arc of movement between 70° and 120° of abduction. Compression may also occur beneath the acromioclavicular joint itself, which may cause a painful arc of movement during the last 30° of abduction, or deep to the coracoacromial ligament [2].

The original version of the chapter has been revised. Keith Diamond has been removed from the author group. A correction to this chapter can be found at https://doi.org/10.1007/978-3-030-80402-2_11

M. A. Hemida (✉)
Orthopedic Surgery, Ain Shams University, Cairo, Egypt

K. Zhai · D. King · J. Genin
Department of Orthopedic Surgery, Cleveland Clinic Foundation, Cleveland, OH, USA

11

Impingement can often then progress to further degenerative shoulder pathology. Impingement involves abutment of the hypertrophied cuff tendon with the undersurface of the acromion, which can sometimes also involve other pathology such as a subacromial spur or acromioclavicular arthritis. If neglected or mis-treated, impingement can lead to degeneration, rotator cuff arthropathy, and even a rotator cuff tear [2].

3.2 History

Precise history taking is a critical component in working up and diagnosing patients with a shoulder complaint. The following are some important considerations when conducting a patient history [3].

Age. Degenerative shoulder diseases usually occur in the **elderly** although it may occur in young athletes. It may also occur in anyone who repeatedly performs overhead throwing motions, as the recurrent friction between the tendon and/or the bursa with the undersurface of the acromion. Shoulder instability, on the other hand, is more common in **young** patients. These patients often have a lax capsule and are more susceptible to injuries as a result [4].

Pain. The most common cause of shoulder pain is cervical spondylosis. Pain or irritation of nerve roots in the neck is referred to the shoulder. Complaints of anterolateral shoulder pain ("over the Codman zone") are often suggestive of degenerative shoulder pathology such as impingement or rotator cuff tear, especially if accompanied by night pain. Biceps tendinitis, on the other hand, typically causes deeper anterior shoulder pain, which can also be caused by subcoracoid impingement and more medial bursitis [4].

Stiffness. In patients who complain of limited ROM due to pain, impingement or rotator cuff tear is often the underlying cause. Other causes of stiffness could be arthritis and frozen shoulder, i.e., *adhesive capsulitis* [4].

Instability. In the case of instability, it is important to ask the following questions. The answers to these questions can help narrow the differential and provide some clarity on whether the patient may have a glenohumeral bony defect and poor soft tissue quality.

- When was the first time of dislocation?
- Was the dislocation an anterior or posterior dislocation?
- What was the mechanism of dislocation?
- How many times has the patient dislocated their shoulder?
- Was the dislocation reduced by the patient themselves or in a hospital?
- If in a hospital, was the dislocation reduced under general anesthesia? [3, 4].

Occupation. Manual workers (e.g., carpenters) as well as overhead athletes (e.g., baseball players) are more likely to suffer from impingement syndrome [4].

Medical History. Patients with a history of diabetes or hypothyroidism are at a higher risk of developing frozen shoulder. Patients with epilepsy often suffer from recurrent shoulder dislocation. For these patients, surgical management may be an option, but the seizures must be well-controlled with no seizures for 3 months prior to surgery [3].

Surgical History. Patients with a history of a proximal humerus fracture or mal-united greater tuberosity have a greater risk of suffering from impingement disease [3, 4].

3.3   Examination

Inspection. A virtual inspection includes assessment for swelling, muscle wasting, or scars from any previous operations. Anteriorly, the physician can assess for the presence of (a) prominent sternoclavicular joint (*subluxation*), (b) deformity of clavicle (*old fracture*), (c) prominent acromioclavicular joint (*subluxation or osteo-arthritis*), and (d) deltoid wasting (*disuse or axillary nerve palsy*) (Fig. 3.1). Laterally, the physician can observe for swelling of the joint, suggesting an infectious or inflammatory reaction, which could suggest an underlying etiology of cal-cifying supraspinatus tendinitis, pyrogenic infection of the glenohumeral joint, or trauma (Fig. 3.2). Posteriorly, the physician should inspect the scapula for shape and position. Small and high scapulae may suggest Sprengel's shoulder or Klippel-Feil syndrome. The physician should also look for any signs of webbing of skin at the root of the neck and winging of the scapula, which may suggest paralysis of the ser-ratus anterior [3–5] (Fig. 3.3).

Range of Motion. Active ROM assessment can be completed by performing the appropriate motions and instructing the patient to repeat the motion while asking for the presence of pain, which is especially important during shoulder abduction. It is important to ask the patient to perform external rotation in both adduction and abduction. If external rotation is limited especially in comparison to the other side, this may suggest frozen shoulder. Normal values for shoulder ROM include

Fig. 3.1 Inspection from the front

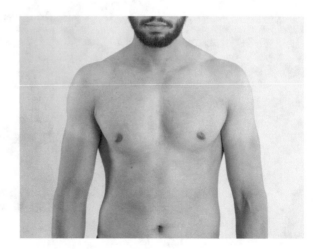

Fig. 3.2 Inspection from
the side

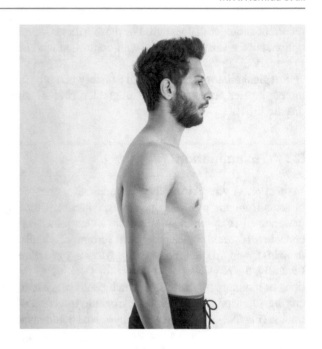

Fig. 3.3 Inspection from
the back

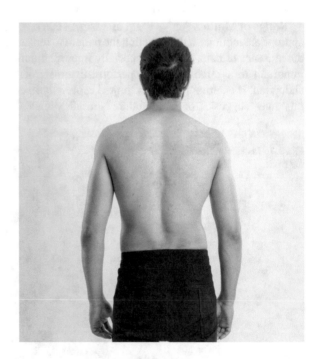

Fig. 3.4 90° shoulder abduction

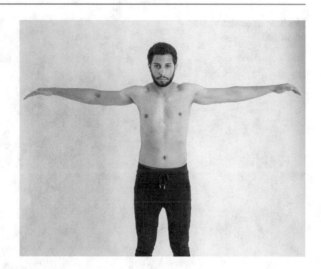

Fig. 3.5 Maximum shoulder abduction

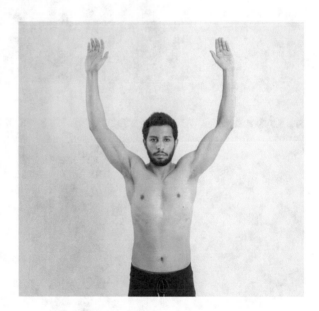

abduction up to 150° (Figs. 3.4 and 3.5), adduction up to 30–50° (Fig. 3.6), flexion from 0° to 180° (Figs. 3.7 and 3.8), extension from 0° to 60° (Fig. 3.9), external rotation up to 90° (Figs. 3.10, 3.11, and 3.12), and internal rotation up to 70–90° [4, 5] (Figs. 3.11, 3.12, and 3.13).

Special Test: Impingement Assessment. Ask the patient to forward flex their shoulder, flex their elbow to 90°, and then internally rotate their shoulder. If this elicits pain mostly in the lateral and anterolateral shoulder region, the test is positive and suggests impingement [5] (Figs. 3.14 and 3.15).

Fig. 3.6 Shoulder adduction

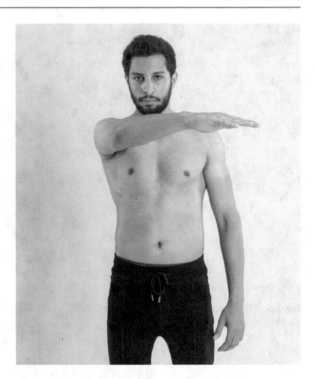

Fig. 3.7 90° Shoulder flexion

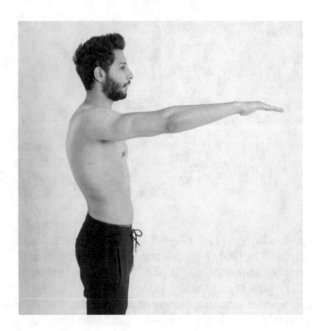

Fig. 3.8 Maximum
shoulder flexion

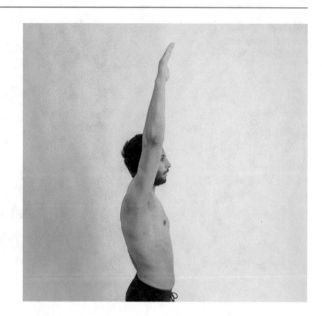

Fig. 3.9 Shoulder
extension

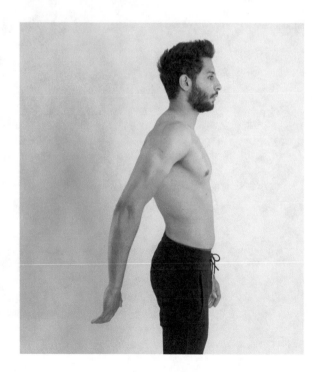

Fig. 3.10 Shoulder
external rotation in
adduction

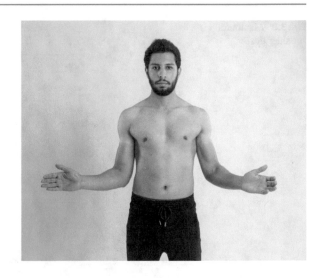

Fig. 3.11 Shoulder
internal rotation in
adduction

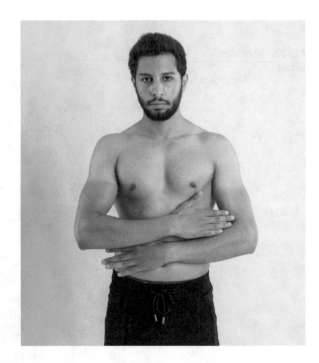

Fig. 3.12 Shoulder
external rotation in
abduction

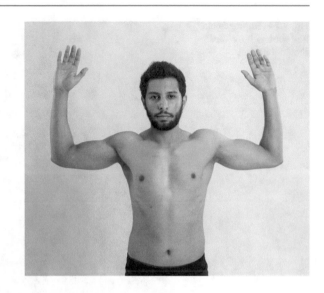

Fig. 3.13 Shoulder
internal rotation in
abduction

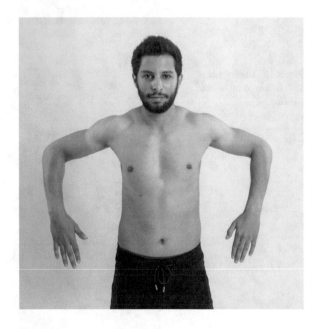

Fig. 3.14 Impingement test: start with forward shoulder flexion

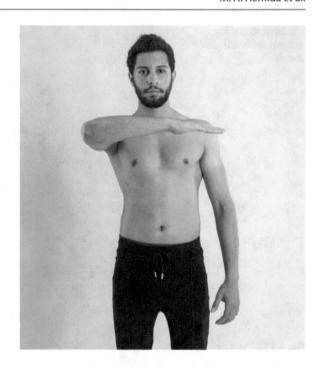

Fig. 3.15 Impingement test: followed by internal rotation

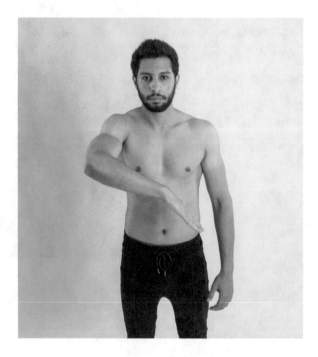

3.4   Resisted Abduction Test

Equipment required: Any item weights 2 kg.

Ask the patient to do shoulder abduction while he is lifting 2 kg object with shoulder internal rotation. This test simulates empty can test for rotator cuff tear [4] (Figs. 3.16 and 3.17).

Special Test: Modified Empty Can Test. An approximately 2-kg weighted object is required as an additional piece of equipment. For this test, ask the patient to perform shoulder abduction while lifting the 2-kg object and with the

Fig. 3.16 Modified empty can test

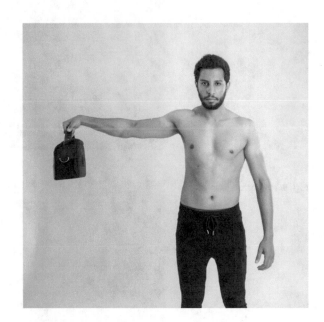

Fig. 3.17 Empty can test

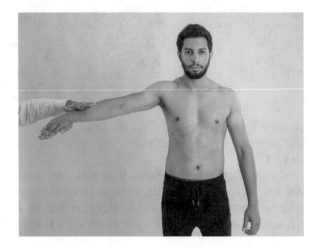

Fig. 3.18 Modified
speed test

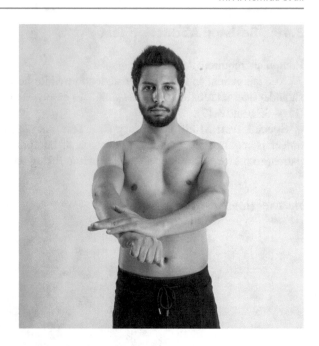

Fig. 3.19 Speed test

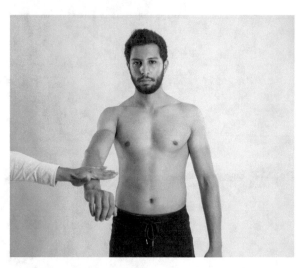

shoulder internally rotated. This test is a virtual adaptation of the empty can test and suggests a rotator cuff tear if the movement elicits pain [4, 5] (Figs. 3.16 and 3.17).

Special Test: Modified Speed Test. Ask the patient to forward flex their shoulder with forearm in pronation while resisting the movement with the other hand over the forearm. This test is a virtual adaptation of the speed test, and pain indicates a positive test and suggests a SLAP lesion [5] (Figs. 3.18 and 3.19).

Fig. 3.20 Modified apprehension test

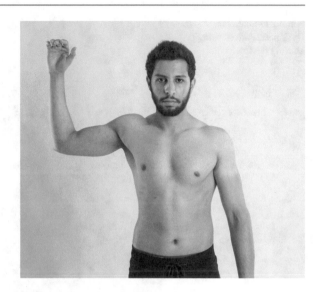

Special Test: Modified Apprehension Test. Ask the patient to abduct their shoulder to 90° and externally rotate to 90° and ask the patient whether they feel worried that the shoulder might dislocate. This test is a virtual adaptation of the apprehension test for anterior shoulder instability [6] (Fig. 3.20).

Special Test: Scapular Dyskinesia Assessment. Ask the patient to forward flex the shoulder while inspecting their back to follow scapular motion. Monitor the symmetry of scapular motion during this movement [6] (Figs. 3.21 and 3.22).

Special Test: Scapular Winging Assessment. Instruct the patient to lean with both hands against a wall. Watch the inferior angle of the scapula for any winging [5] (Figs. 3.23 and 3.24).

3.5 Radiology

Plain Film X-Ray (PXR). The **AP and scapular Y view** can be used to assess the acromion morphology. A type B or type C hooked acromion may cause impingement. PXR also aids to exclude the presence of arthritis or proximal migration as in rotator cuff arthropathy, or disuse osteopenia which may occur in the case frozen shoulder. The **supraspinatus outlet view** allows classification of the acromion morphology as well. In the **Zanca view**, the AC joint can be visualized to reveal any pathology such as AC joint disease or distal clavicle osteolysis. The **Stryker Notch view** can be used to detect a Hill-Sachs lesion. The **West Point view** can be used to assess for anteroinferior glenoid, bony Bankart, or proximal humerus fracture. Finally, the **Serendipity view** can be used to assess for anterior and posterior sternoclavicular dislocation [6, 7].

Computer Tomography (CT). Compared with PXR, the CT modality offers better assessment of bony defects and magnification artifacts that are associated

Fig. 3.21 Scapular
Dyskinesia Assessment.
Starting flexion

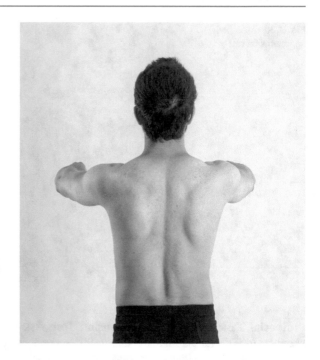

Fig. 3.22 Scapular
Dyskinesia Assessment:
maximum forward flexion

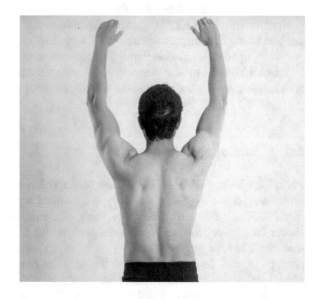

with radiographs do not occur with CT. CT also provides better detail of cortical and
trabecular bone structures than magnetic resonance imaging (MRI) at the cost of
higher radiation exposure. **Axial shoulder images** are useful for visualizing Reverse
Hill-Sachs lesions. **Sagittal shoulder images** can be useful for visualizing

Fig. 3.23 Scapular Winging Assessment (side view)

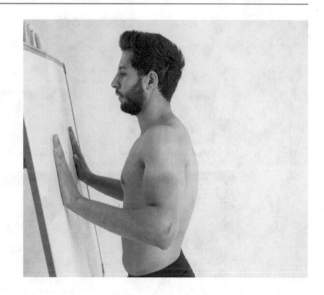

Fig. 3.24 Scapular Winging Assessment (back view)

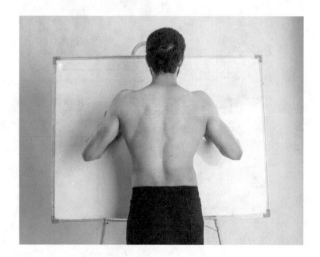

anterior-inferior glenoid insufficiency. Finally, **3D reconstructions** can be useful for visualizing glenoid defects [6].

Magnetic Resonance Imaging (MRI). MRI is best for evaluating soft tissue structures and evaluation bone contusions or trabecular microfractures. It can be an especially useful radiographic modality for the assessment of rotator cuff integrity, biceps tendon integrity, subacromial bursitis, or AC arthritis. Additionally, the **MR arthrogram** is commonly used to augment MRI studies to diagnose soft-tissue problems such as SLAP tears [7].

The following mind map helps to approach shoulder assessment via telemedicine (Fig. 3.25).

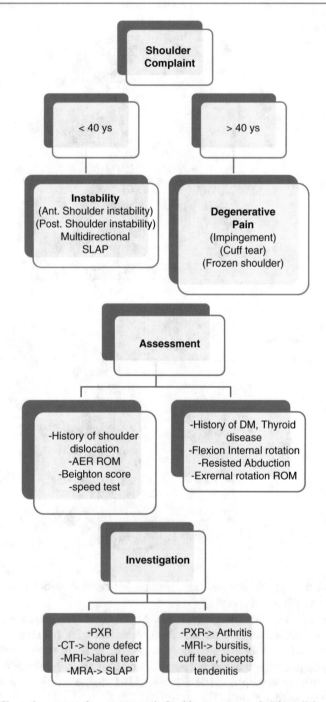

Fig. 3.25 Charts demonstrate how to approach shoulder assessment via telemedicine

References

1. Farber JM, Buckwalter KA. Sports-related injuries of the shoulder: instability. Radiol Clin. 2002;40(2):235–49.
2. Daruwalla ZJ, Wong KL, Thambiah J. The application of telemedicine in orthopedic surgery in Singapore: a pilot study on a secure, mobile telehealth application and messaging platform. JMIR Mhealth Uhealth. 2014;2(2):e28.
3. McFarland EG, Kibler WB, Murrell GA, Rojas J. Examination of the shoulder for beginners and experts: an update. Instr Course Lect. 2020;69:255–72.
4. McRae R. Clinical orthopaedic examination. London: Churchill Livingstone/Elsevier; 2010.
5. Lazaro LE, Cordasco FA. Physical exam of the adolescent shoulder: tips for evaluating and diagnosing common shoulder disorders in the adolescent athlete. Curr Opin Pediatr. 2017;29(1):70–9.
6. Colak C, Winalski CS. Fundamentals in shoulder radiology. In: Shoulder arthroplasty. Cham: Springer; 2020. p. 123–40.
7. Akel I, Pekmezci M, Hayran M, Genc Y, Kocak O, Derman O, Erdoğan I, Yazici M. Evaluation of shoulder balance in the normal adolescent population and its correlation with radiological parameters. Eur Spine J. 2008;17(3):348–54.

Elbow and Forearm

4

Mostafa Gemeah, Keith Diamond, Mitchell Ng, and Peter Evans

4.1 Overview

The elbow joint is a complex joint formed by three bones: the distal part of the humerus, the olecranon, and the radial head. The joint is surrounded by a capsule and supported by both lateral and medial collateral ligaments that help provide joint stability during motion. Elbow flexion is mediated by the biceps, brachialis, and brachioradialis muscles. Extension is mediated by the three-headed triceps muscle. Through contraction of these muscles, elbow movement plays an important role in the function of the hand by controlling the functional length of the upper limb and acting as a lever arm. The elbow joint is surrounded by important nerves (*ulnar nerve, radial nerve, medial nerve, musculocutaneous nerve*) that are responsible for motor and sensory innervation of the forearm and hand [1, 2].

There are many diagnostic methods in the evaluation of the elbow that can be easily translated to the telemedicine setting. Patient history taking, inspection, and many special tests can all be performed virtually. Taken together, these assessment modalities can be integrated by the surgeon and used to decide which investigations are still necessary for confirming the diagnosis. Fortunately, in the case of the elbow,

The original version of the chapter has been revised. Keith Diamond has been added to the author group. A correction to this chapter can be found at https://doi.org/10.1007/978-3-030-80402-2_11

M. Gemeah
Health Care Innovation Program, Arizona State University, Tempe, AZ, USA
e-mail: mgemeah@asu.edu

K. Diamond · M. Ng
Department of Orthopedic Surgery, Maimonides Medical Center, Brooklyn, NY, USA

P. Evans (✉)
Department of Orthopedic Surgery, Cleveland Clinic Foundation, Cleveland, OH, USA
e-mail: evansp@ccf.org

common pathologies such as arthritis, tendonitis, fractures, and instability are highly amenable to telemedicine assessment and diagnosis.

4.2 History

The history and patient interview can provide significant diagnostic values in the evaluation of elbow pathology. Personal characteristics such as age, surgical history, various symptoms assessments, and the mechanism of injury can all help to guide the surgeon towards the correct diagnosis.

4.2.1 Personal History

Age: Many diseases and fracture types occur with varying frequencies by age group. For example, a pulled elbow (also known as "nursemaid's elbow") is a common injury in children under the age of 5. Arthritis, on the other hand, is much more common with older patients.

Sex: Some elbow pathologies exhibit different incidences among males and females. Rheumatoid arthritis, for example, is more common in the female patients.

Occupation: Occupational laborers who use heavy tools frequently develop lateral epicondylitis. Athletic participation, whether professionally or recreationally, can predispose patients to certain elbow pathologies. Tennis players frequently develop lateral epicondylitis, hence the name *tennis elbow*, while golfers often develop medial epicondylitis, hence *golfer's elbow*. Hand dominance is another consideration; tendinitis of the elbow typically affects the ipsilateral elbow of the dominant hand [3].

Surgical History: Patients with a history of a malunion fracture of the distal humerus may suffer from stiffness and deformity of the elbow [3].

4.2.2 Complain

Mechanism of Injury: If the patient complaint is secondary to trauma, varying mechanisms of injury can suggest specific pathologies. Falls on outstretched hands often result in posterior dislocation, supracondylar fracture, and radial head injury. Direct blows to the elbow can lead to olecranon fracture. Pulling children up by the arm can cause radial head subluxation, leading to a pulled elbow [3, 4].

Pain. Patients with elbow complaints most commonly present with pain. Generalized pain all over the elbow is suggestive of arthritis and can be septic, rheumatoid, or osteoarthritis. Localized pain over the lateral epicondyle is specific for tennis elbow, radial tunnel syndrome, or osteochondritis of the capitulum. Localized pain over the medial epicondyle is specific for golfer's elbow, cubital tunnel syndrome, and ulnar collateral ligament injury. Aching pain suggests arthritic changes. Pain with activity is usually due to tendinosis or instability. Pain may radiate to the mid-humerus and forearm [4].

Stiffness. Stiffness with rest or in the early morning is suggestive of arthritis, especially rheumatoid arthritis or osteoarthritis. Stiffness may also be present following a traumatic malunion or fracture [4].

Swelling. Swelling may be generalized or localized. Generalized swelling is associated with rheumatoid, septic, or osteoarthritis. Localized swelling is often related to rheumatoid nodules, bursitis, and gouty tophi [3, 4].

4.3 Examination

4.3.1 Inspection

Can be done via telemedicine to examine for swelling, muscle wasting or scars of previous operation, deformity. Elbow should be inspected in flexion and extension from all sides. Elbow should be inspected in extension with arm by patient side and forearm supinated for determining carrying angle in males normally about 11° and female normally about 13°. It is increased (cubitus valgus) in case of lateral condyle fracture nonunion and premature lateral epiphysis closure (this usually associated with ulnar nerve palsy) and decreased with supracondylar humerus fracture (Figs. 4.1 and 4.2).

Inspection. Inspection can be performed through a video-enabled virtual platform to assess for swelling, muscle wasting, deformity, or scars from prior operations. The

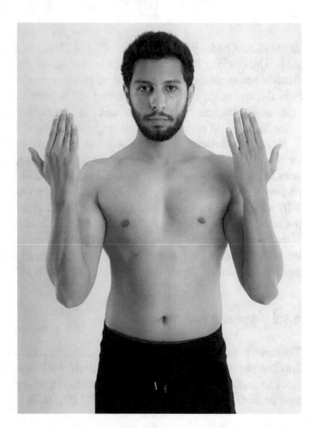

Fig. 4.1 Inspection of the posterior aspect of the elbow

Fig. 4.2 Inspection of the anterior aspect of the elbow and assessment of carrying angle

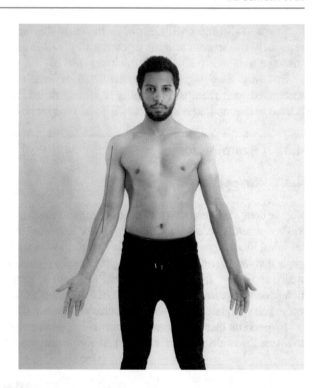

elbow should be inspected in flexion (Fig. 4.1) and in extension (Fig. 4.2) from all sides. The carrying angle can be measured from an anterior view with the patient's shoulders relaxed in anatomical position, elbows extended, and forearms supinated. A typical carrying angle is 11° in males and 13° in females (Fig. 4.2). An increased carrying angle indicates cubitus valgus and can occur in the case of lateral condyle malunion fracture and premature lateral epiphysis closure [3, 4].

Range of Motion. To assess the active ROM, the provider can demonstrate the motion and then ask the patient to repeat. Flexion and extension ROM can be tested with the patient's shoulder by their side using a lateral view. In a typical healthy patient, flexion should be up to 140° (Fig. 4.3) and extension should be down to −10° (Fig. 4.4). Pronation and supination ROM can be tested by instructing the patient to flex their elbows 90° by their side and using an anterior view (Fig. 4.5). Normal pronation is 0–70° (Fig. 4.6) and normal supination is 0–80° (Fig. 4.7). A limited ROM is often found with a history of fracture and arthritis. Bilateral comparison can further narrow the differential diagnosis [4].

4.3.2 Special Tests

Thomsen's Test for Tennis Elbow. The patient should be asked to clench their fist, dorsiflex their wrist, and extend their elbow while another person provides resistance to dorsiflexion. If pain develops over the lateral epicondyle, the test is considered positive and suggests tennis elbow [4] (Fig. 4.8).

Fig. 4.3 Assessing active flexion range of the elbow

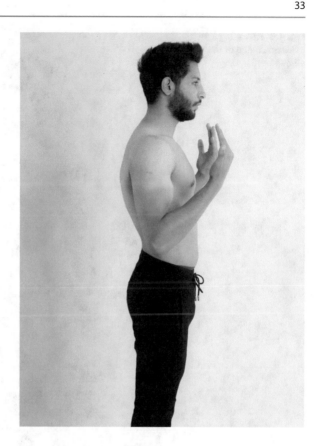

Tinel's Test for Ulnar Nerve Entrapment and Neuropathy. The patient should be asked to flex their elbow to 20°. Another person may then be asked to tap gently between the olecranon and medial epicondyle over the ulnar groove. The test is positive for ulnar neuropathy if the patient has a tingling sensation down the forearm through the ulnar part of the hand [4] (Figs. 4.9 and 4.10).

Test for Golfer's Elbow. The patient is asked to flex their elbow with the forearm supinated. Another person is asked to attempt to extend the elbow against the patient's resistance. The test is considered positive for golfer's elbow if the movement elicits pain over the medial epicondyle [4].

Chair Push-up Test. This test can be used to assess posterolateral rotator instability in cases of complex collateral ligament injury. The patient will begin in a seated position with their hands grasping the arms of the chair. The elbows will be in 90° of flexion, the forearms will be supinated, and the shoulders will be slightly abducted. The patient should be asked to rise from the chair by pushing down and rising slowly. If the movement elicits elbow pain, the test is considered positive [5, 6] (Fig. 4.11).

Other Stability Tests. Other stability tests such as valgus and varus stress tests are not easily translatable to the telemedicine setting. The diagnostic value

Fig. 4.4 Assessing active extension range of the elbow

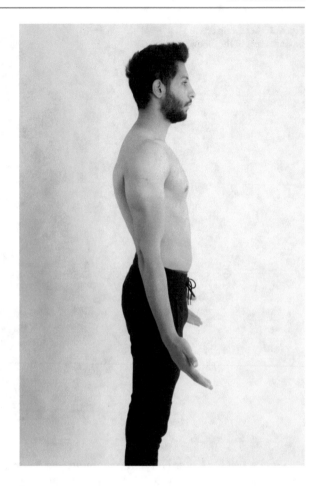

generated by these tests can instead be provided through imaging, especially plain film X-ray (PXR) with stress views [6].

4.4 Investigations

4.4.1 Radiology

Plain Film X-Ray (PXR): PXR is typically indicated for the evaluation of fractures, loose bodies, and the presence of arthritis. AP and lateral views are standard, although other special views may be needed. The internal oblique view is necessary for determining a lateral condyle fracture in children. Stress views are also helpful for assessment of coronal stability [7].

Computer Tomography (CT). This modality is important with traumatic etiologies to show the fracture details needed for development of a specific treatment

Fig. 4.5 Elbow is in
neutral position of
pronation and supination

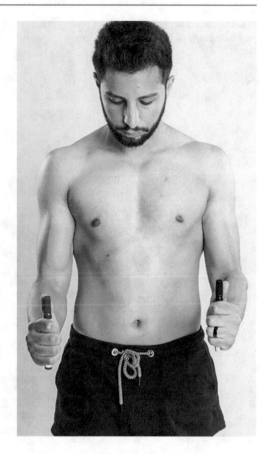

plan. CT is also important for the diagnosis of osteoarthritis and osteochondritis
dissecans [8].

Magnetic Resonance Imaging (MRI). MRI is especially useful in the assessment of soft tissues and can be used to assess the biceps tendons and the triceps
tendons. The medial and lateral collateral ligaments can also be studied using MRI
in cases of instability or cases where there is a history of elbow dislocation.

4.5   Other Investigations

Nerve Conduction Test. This can be used for evaluation of nerve entrapment.

4.5.1   Algorithm for Elbow and Forearm Assessment

This algorithm is a mind map for simplifying the approach of elbow and forearm
problems according to patient complain and virtual assessment of elbow and forearm (Fig. 4.12).

Fig. 4.6 Assessing active pronation range of the elbow

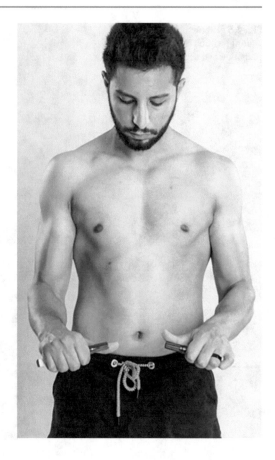

Fig. 4.7 Assessing active supination range of the elbow

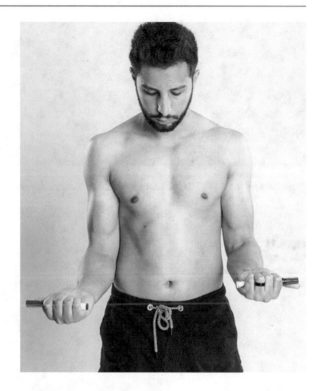

Fig. 4.8 Thomsen's test for tennis elbow diagnosis

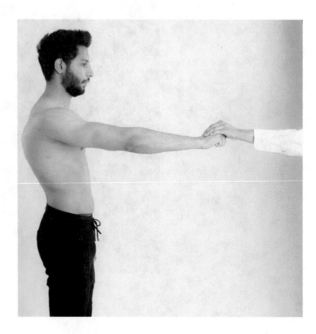

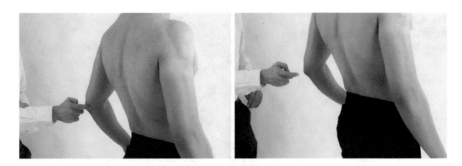

Figs. 4.9 and 4.10 Tinel's test for assessment of ulnar entrapment

Fig. 4.11 Chair push-up test for posterolateral rotatory instability assessment

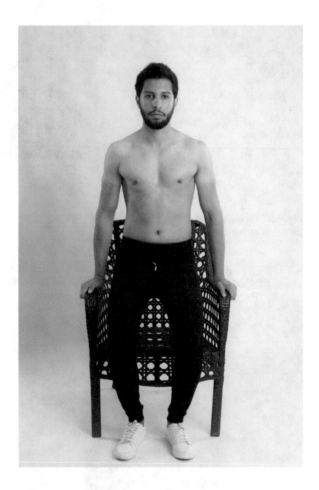

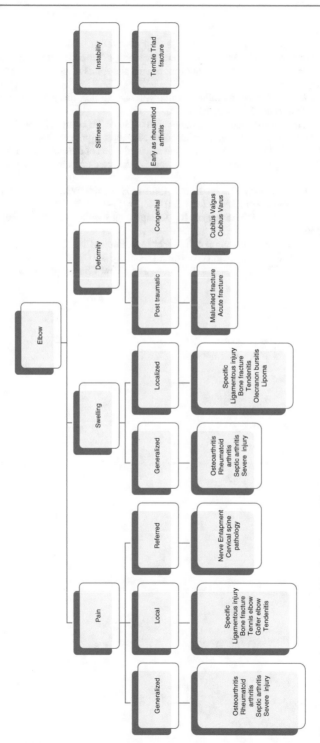

Fig. 4.12 Chart shows an algorithm for elbow and forearm assessment

References

1. Bain G, van den Bekerom M, Mehta JA. Clinical anatomy of the elbow. In: Bain G, Eygendaal D, van Riet R, editors. Surgical techniques for trauma and sports related injuries of the elbow. Berlin: Springer; 2020.
2. Karbach LE, Elfar J. Elbow instability: anatomy, biomechanics, diagnostic maneuvers, and testing. J Hand Surg Am. 2017;42(2):118–26.
3. Chouhan DK, Arjun RHH, Behera P. Examination of elbow. In: Dhatt S, Prabhakar S, editors. Handbook of clinical examination in orthopedics. Singapore: Springer; 2019.
4. Lazinski M, Lazinski M, Fedorczyk JM. Clinical examination of the elbow. In: Rehabilitation of the hand and upper extremity, E-Book, vol. 12. Amsterdam: Elsevier Health Sciences; 2020. p. 76.
5. Anakwenze OA, Kancherla VK, Iyengar J, Ahmad CS, Levine WN. Posterolateral rotatory instability of the elbow. Am J Sports Med. 2014;42(2):485–91.
6. Tarassoli P, McCann P, Amirfeyz R. Complex instability of the elbow. Injury. 2017;48(3):568–77.
7. Guglielmi G, Bazzocchi A. Imaging of the upper limb. Radiol Clin N Am. 2019;57(5):xv.
8. Facchini G, Bazzocchi A, Spinnato P, Albisinni U. CT and 3D CT of the elbow. In: Porcellini G, Rotini R, Stignani KS, Di Giacomo S, editors. The elbow. Cham: Springer; 2018.

Hand and Wrist

5

Shady Abdelghaffar Mahmoud, Ahmed K. Emara, and Joseph Styron

5.1 History

5.1.1 Personal History

Age. The patient's age can provide diagnostic clues, as many hand pathologies are associated with specific age groups. In general, hand pathologies are especially common in the elderly population, with a 20% prevalence of hand pain and 25% prevalence of hand disability [1]. The rate of nerve regeneration in nerve injuries is also affected by age, which may impact surgical treatment and prognosis (Fig. 5.1).

Occupation. The patient's occupation and specific hand movements associated with their occupation provide important context for possible areas of concern. Other considerations such as **handedness** or involvement in **sports** that impact the patient's daily routine activities are important not only for diagnosis, but also for determining a treatment plan that will align with the patient's daily needs [2].

Mechanism of Injury. A traumatic mechanism may result in fractures or sprains. Repetitive use, on the other hand, is more closely associated with neuritis and tendonitis. The type of injury and the timeline are also important in treatment: a knife injury, for example, is treated very differently from a chemical burn.

S. A. Mahmoud
Orthopedic Surgery, Ain Shams University, Cairo, Egypt

A. K. Emara (✉) · J. Styron
Department of Orthopedic Surgery, Cleveland Clinic Foundation, Cleveland, OH, USA

© The Author(s), under exclusive license to Springer Nature Switzerland AG 2022
K. M. Emara, N. S. Piuzzi (eds.), *The Principles of Virtual Orthopedic Assessment*,
https://doi.org/10.1007/978-3-030-80402-2_5

Fig. 5.1 Tools and
equipment to be prepared
for proper virtual hand
assessment

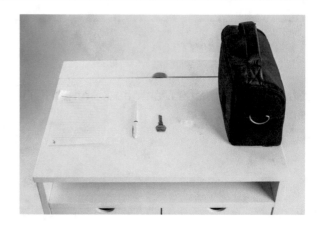

5.1.2   Past History

Medical History. A history of diseases such as rheumatoid arthritis or tuberculosis can be suggestive of particular diagnoses and underlying etiologies. Some systemic diseases such as diabetes mellitus, thyroid disease, and renal diseases are associated with carpal tunnel syndrome.

   Surgical History. Surgery can be the cause of nerve injury, so this can provide diagnostic value. For example, radial nerve injury can be a complication following open reduction and internal fixation of a humerus fracture. Surgical history can also provide context around possible difficulties in any future surgeries and can thus impact treatment planning as well.

   Medications. Especially when working with a new patient, inquiring about medications can often reveal aspects of medical history a patient may not recall or mention. A history of steroid intake, for example, is often associated with rheumatoid arthritis. The use of analgesics, as well as its frequency of use, can also provide additional context around the severity of symptoms [3].

   Family History. Many congenital conditions of the hand have a genetic component. Autosomal dominant conditions include Madelung's deformity, congenital radioulnar synostosis, cleft hand, symphalangism, and syndactyly [3].

5.1.3   Complain

Pain. Hand and wrist pain are very common, with reported prevalence between 3% and 26% of the general population. The specific features of the pain symptoms can provide significant diagnostic value. Most importantly, the **site** of the pain can suggest which anatomical structures are involved. Ulnar side wrist pain can suggest a triangular fibrocartilage complex (TFCC) tear, distal radioulnar joint instability or arthritis, pisotriquetral arthritis, extensor carpi ulnaris instability, or a hamate fracture. Radial side wrist pain may suggest De Quervain's tendonitis [4], a scaphoid fracture [5, 6], scapho-trapezio-triquetral arthritis, basilar thumb carpometacarpal arthritis, or scapholunate instability [7]. Pain along the course of a certain nerve with accompanying symptoms like tingling, numbness, or paresthesia is suggestive of nerve injury. Pain that follows a dermatomal distribution, on the other hand, is more suggestive of radicular nerve root compression. A sudden **onset** of pain is typically more suggestive of mechanical factors or a traumatic injury. Pain that is **aggravated** by activities and **relieved** by rest can suggest arthritis. By contrast, pain secondary to neoplastic or infectious etiologies is often more constant, or nocturnal. Pain that is aggravated by specific motions, e.g., opening a jar, can also point to specific anatomical defects. The **intensity** of the pain can also be assessed, using a subjective 1–10-point pain scale or by inquiring about the impact on daily activities like work or sleep patterns.

Stiffness. Stiffness that lasts more than half an hour, especially in the morning, may indicate an inflammatory etiology and is suggestive of rheumatoid arthritis.

Swelling. Swelling can also suggest inflammation, although it is associated with fractures and tumors as well. Painless, slow-growing swelling at the dorsum of the hand just distal to the lister tubercle is suggestive of a ganglion cyst. These may also present as occult ganglion cysts, which are associated with pain but no swelling.

Deformity. Wrist drop can suggest a radial nerve injury while a partial claw hand suggests ulnar nerve involvement. More severe claw deformities are associated with more distal levels of involvement with the ulnar nerve, a phenomenon known as the *ulnar paradox*.

Lack of Dexterity. This may indicate local conditions such as thumb carpometacarpal arthritis, regional conditions such as nerve injury, or general conditions such as myelopathy.

Other Symptoms. Other relevant symptoms include weakness, instability, and any mechanical symptoms such as clicking, snapping, catching, popping, and locking. If the problem occurs bilaterally or if other joints like the elbow and shoulder are involved, rheumatoid arthritis is more likely. Constitutional symptoms like fever, nocturnal sweating, generalized pain, and cachexia may indicate an infectious etiology [3].

5.2 Examination

Inspection. A great deal of hand diseases can be observed directly through inspection. To provide a full examination of the hand and wrist, the patient's arms should be relaxed and exposed up to the shoulder. The patient's elbow should fall naturally by their side, with hands placed comfortably on a table (Fig. 5.2). Both hands should be inspected simultaneously to allow for comparison. The hand should be inspected from the dorsal, volar, and lateral angles (Figs. 5.2, 5.3, and 5.4). Begin by observing the general **shape** and **size** of the hand relative to the rest of the patient. Short, stumpy fingers may suggest achondroplasia. Large and coarse fingers may suggest acromegaly. Hypertrophy of the finger can suggest Paget disease, neurofibromatosis, or a local arteriovenous fistula.

Fig. 5.2 Exposure needed for hand assessment

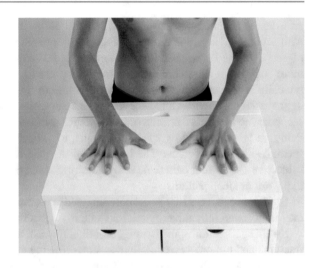

Fig. 5.3 Inspect the volar surface of the hand

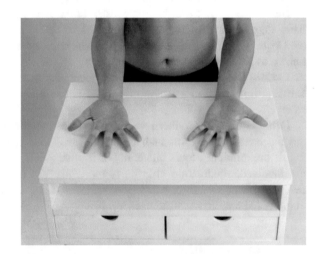

Fig. 5.4 Inspect the sides of the hand with extended thumb and fingers

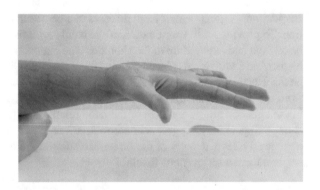

Next, observe the **nails** for any disturbance of growth, deformity, or evidence of fungal infection or psoriasis. The **skin** may also provide diagnostic clues, and it is important to look for the presence of finger burns or trophic ulceration that may be suggestive of neurological disturbance. Any alteration in skin color may suggest circulatory involvement. Any dryness in the skin may be associated with myxedema. Scars should be noted as well.

Moving on to the muscles around the hand and wrist, note any **muscle wasting** that can suggest a root, plexus, or nerve lesion. For example, wasting at the thenar eminence may indicate median nerve injury while wasting of the hypothenar and interossei muscles may indicate a distal ulnar nerve injury. If the hypothenar wasting is associated with additional involvement of the volar distal ulnar forearm, a more proximal ulnar nerve injury is possible. Wasting at the anatomical snuff box may indicate radial nerve injury.

Next, observe the wrist for any **swelling**. The most common causes of swelling include collateral ligament tears, rheumatoid nodules, osteoarthritis, and ganglion cysts. Other less common causes include tuberculosis, gout, and psoriatic arthritis. Heberden's node at the dorsum of the distal interphalangeal (DIP) joint and Bouchard node at the proximal interphalangeal (PIP) joint are classically swellings associated with arthritis [3].

Finally, observe for any characteristic **deformities** in the hand, many of which are specific to various pathologies. A flexed DIP joint in isolation can suggest mallet finger. Other deformities can be associated with varying pathologies. These include swan neck deformities characterized by flexion at the DIP and hyperextension at the PIP joint, Boutonniere deformities characterized by flexion at the PIP and extension at the DIP joint, and Z-deformities of the thumb characterized by flexion at the metacarpophalangeal (MP) and extension at the interphalangeal (IP) joints. Congenital flexion or coronal deformity of the little finger is caused by congenital contracture and is called camptodactyly and clinodactyly, respectively. Flexion of a finger at the MP joint suggests traumatic extensor injury when associated with loss of active extension. Flexion at the MP joint may also suggest Dupuytren's contracture if it involves multiple fingers and is also associated with IP joint flexion and pea-like nodular thickening in the palm and along the tendon sheath of the finger. Flexion of the PIP joint with a history of clicking and locking suggests trigger finger, especially if there is a nodule on the corresponding MP joint. Clawing of the thumb and fingers with forearm wasting is suggesting of Volkmann's ischemic contracture. Flexion of the fingers at the MP joint with extension at the IP joint may suggest ischemic contracture of small muscles of the hand. Rheumatoid arthritis is also associated with specific deformities including ulnar deviation of the fingers at the MP joint, zigzag hand deformity, dorsal ulnar head prominence, and other finger deformities [8].

Palpation. Although palpation cannot be assessed directly by the provider in a telemedicine visit, the patient can be instructed to indicate possible sites of pain using a black marker. This method provides an indirect way of assessing tenderness. Alternatively, the patient can be provided labeled anatomical diagrams and asked to apply pressure to the indicated areas in an attempt to elicit tenderness (Figs. 5.5 and 5.6).

Fig. 5.5 Front view map to guide the patient where to press to elicit tenderness. 1: Carpometacarpal joint of the thumb, 2: scaphoid tubercle, 3: styloid radius, 4: distal radius, 5: Flexor carpi radialis tendon, 6: Palmaris longus, 7: Flexor carpi ulnaris tendon, 8: pisiform bone, 9: hook of hamate bone, 10: triangular fibrocartilage ligament

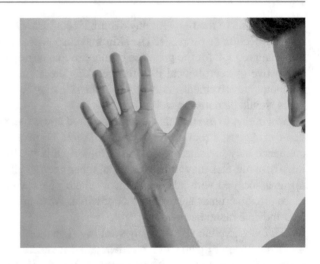

Fig. 5.6 Back view map to guide the patient where to press to elicit tenderness. 1: anatomical snuff box, 2: lister tubercle, 3: scapholunate ligament, 4: radioulnar joint, 5: head ulna, 6: extensor digitorum tendon, 7: adductor pollicis muscle, 8: extensor pollicis longus tendon, 9: base of fifth metacarpal bone

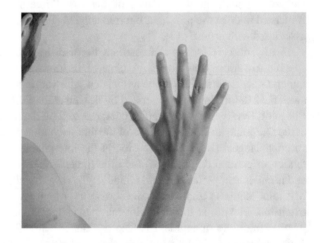

Range of Motion. Active range of motion (ROM) assessment can be readily translated to the telemedicine setting. The use of well-designed software tools (see Chap. 2) can allow for accurate assessment and documentation of ROM for both clinical follow-up and future research purposes.

Testing can begin with assessment of **composite movement** involving grasping and holding with involvement of all finger joints. This assessment can be performed by asking the patient to make a fist with forearms supinated (Fig. 5.7) and pronated (Fig. 5.8). Both hands are assessed simultaneously to allow for comparison. Normally, all distal phalanges should be touching the palm. Any reductions in composite finger flexion ROM can be quantified by measuring the fingertip-to-palm distance using a ruler [3].

Each finger joint can then be **individually tested**. To begin, each finger can be flexed maximally while other fingers remain extended (Fig. 5.9) and then extended

Fig. 5.7 Screening composite movement with palm up

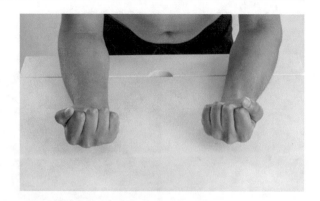

Fig. 5.8 Screening composite movement with palm down

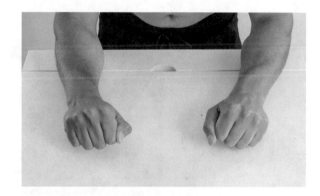

Fig. 5.9 Finger joints flexion range

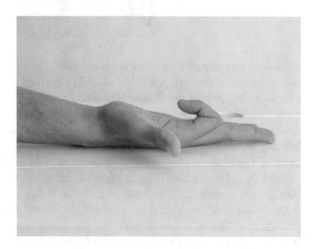

maximally (Fig. 5.4). Static images can be taken from the sagittal view using built-in telemedicine software capabilities or a simple screen capture function, allowing for more precise virtual goniometer measurement. (See Chap. 2 for a list of goniometer software applications.) The **thumbs** can then be assessed for ROM in flexion,

Fig. 5.10 Thumb flexion range

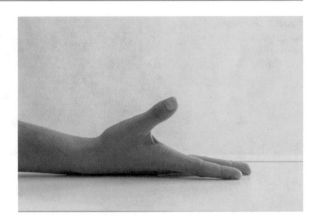

Fig. 5.11 Thumb palmar abduction range

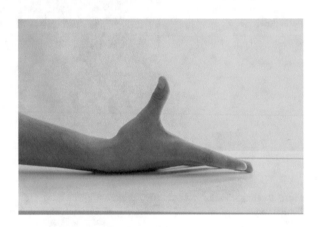

extension, and palmar abduction, applying virtual goniometry as well for more precise measurements (Figs. 5.4, 5.10, and 5.11). Normal active ROM is 0–90° for the MP joint, 0–100° for the PIP joint, 0–80° for the DIP joint, −20° to 15° for the thumb carpometacarpal (CMC) joint, and −20° to 80° for the thumb IP joint. **Wrist** flexion and extension can be assessed with a sagittal view (Figs. 5.12 and 5.13). Moving the camera higher to provide a more oblique sagittal view allows for assessment of finger abduction and adduction (Figs. 5.14 and 5.15), thumb adduction, abduction, and opposition (Figs. 5.16, 5.17, and 5.18), wrist ulnar and radial deviation (Figs. 5.19 and 5.20), and wrist supination and pronation (Figs. 5.21, 5.22, and 5.23). For each of these ROM assessments, the virtual goniometer can be applied to provide quantitative measurements. An alternative method for quantification is to measure distances using a ruler: distance between thumb and little finger for limited opposition, distance between thumb tip and the transverse palmar crease for limited thumb adduction, and distance between the index and little fingers for finger abduction.

Fig. 5.12 Wrist flexion range

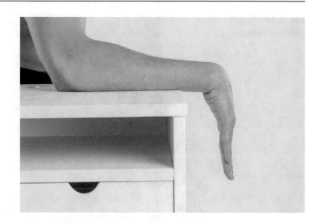

Fig. 5.13 Wrist extension range

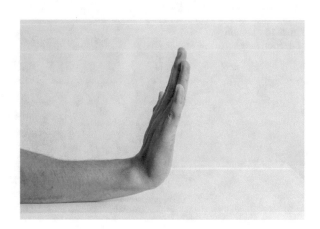

Fig. 5.14 Fingers abduction range

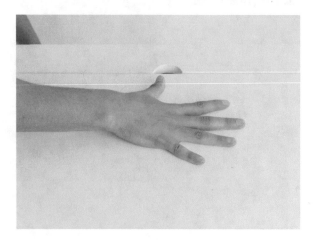

Fig. 5.15 Fingers
adduction range

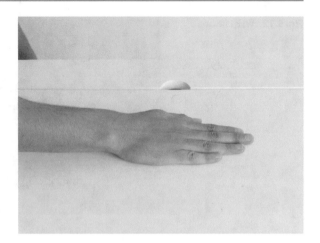

Fig. 5.16 Thumb
adduction range

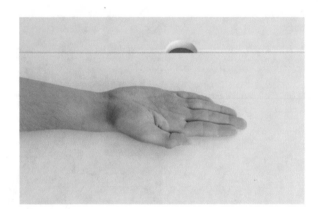

Fig. 5.17 Thumb radial
abduction range

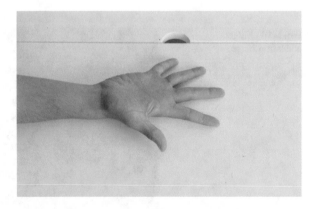

Fig. 5.18 Thumb opposition range

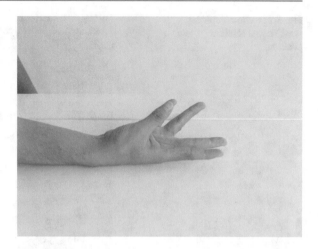

Fig. 5.19 Wrist ulnar deviation range

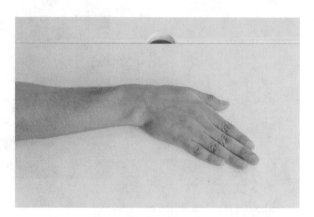

Fig. 5.20 Wrist radial deviation range

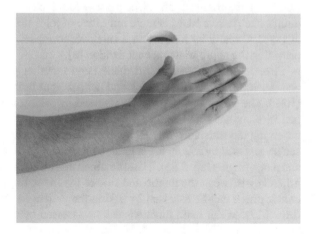

Fig. 5.21 Photo depicts
wrist neutral rotation
position

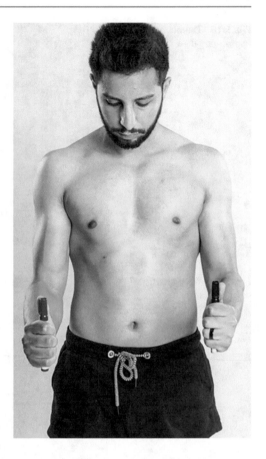

Although **passive ROM** can be more difficult to assess virtually, it is of critical diagnostic value especially in the presence of limited active ROM. When active ROM is compromised, an intact passive ROM can suggest tendon injury while diminished passive ROM is more indicative of joint stiffness. These motions can be assessed virtually by instructing a caregiver to repeat the active ROM tests while providing the appropriate manual fixation [9].

Functional Assessment. Adequate hand function primarily depends on grasp and pinch (90%), while the hook and paperweight function are minor contributors (10%). The **grasp** function can be assessed by asking the patient to firmly grasp a pen in their hand and asking a caregiver to attempt to withdraw the pen while observing the resistance offered by the patient (Fig. 5.24). The **end pinch** function can be assessed by asking the patient to pick up a pen between the tips of the thumb and index finger (Fig. 5.25). The **side pinch** can be assessed by asking the patient to grip a key between the thumb and side of the index finger (Fig. 5.26). Finally, the **chuck pinch** can be assessed by asking the patient to pick up a coin on the table (Fig. 5.27). Minor hand functions can be assessed by asking the patient to carry a

Fig. 5.22 Wrist
supination range

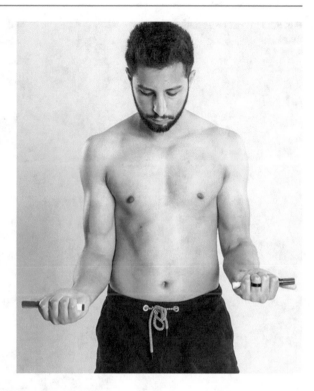

weighted bag to test the **hook** function (Fig. 5.28) and hold a book by their palm to
test the **paperweight** function (Fig. 5.29) [9].

Neurological Assessment. Although neurological assessment is important in the
context of nerve injuries, it does not translate readily to the telemedicine setting.

To conduct **sensory assessment**, a caregiver will need to be present with the
patient and be provided charts indicating the five particular hand regions that will
need to be stimulated using cotton. These regions (and the nerve injuries they are
designed to assess) include: the tip of the index finger (distal median nerve injury),
the thenar eminence (proximal median nerve injury), the tip of the little finger (distal ulnar nerve injury), the hypothenar eminence (proximal ulnar nerve injury)
(Fig. 5.30), and the snuff box region (radial nerve injury) (Fig. 5.31). If the diagnosis is still in question following these virtual assessments, a face-to-face visit or
nerve conduction velocity test will be required to establish a final diagnosis [10].

For **motor assessment**, begin by asking the patient to make an "OK" sign with
the tips of their thumb and index finger. Then, if there is a caregiver present, ask
them to provide resistance and attempt to break the "O." Failure to complete the "O"
or weakness to resistance may indicate an interosseous nerve injury (Figs. 5.32 and
5.33). Next, the strength of active wrist extension can be assessed. If the patient
demonstrates a wrist drop or is unable to fully extend their wrist against gravity,
there may be a radial nerve injury or a posterior interosseous nerve (PIN) injury if
accompanied by radial deviation. Additional pain in the dorsum of the forearm

Fig. 5.23 Wrist pronation range

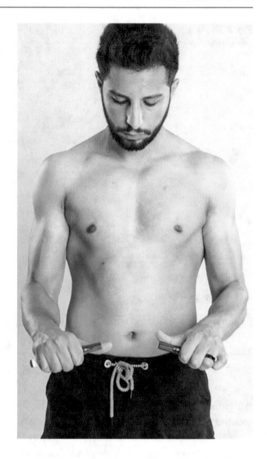

Fig. 5.24 Grasp hand function

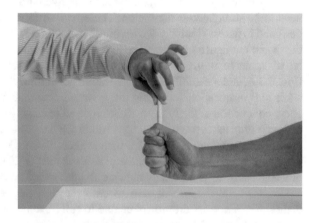

Fig. 5.25 End pinch hand function

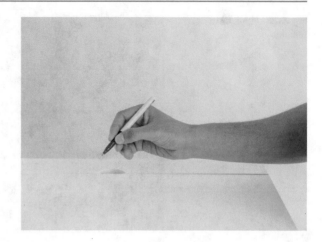

Fig. 5.26 Side pinch hand function

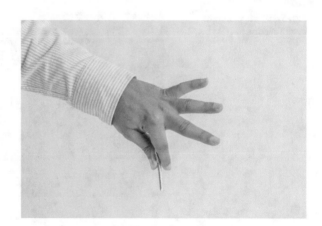

Fig. 5.27 Chuck pinch hand function

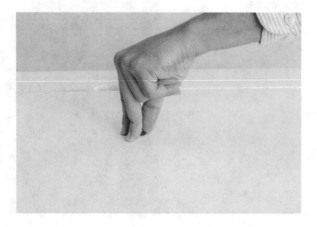

Fig. 5.28 Hook hand
function

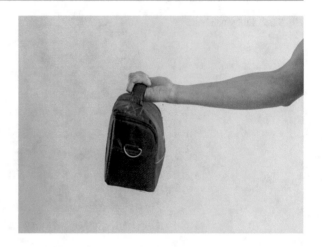

Fig. 5.29 Paperweight
hand function

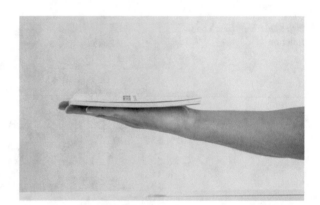

Fig. 5.30 Hand chart
from the front
demonstrates the sites of
sensory assessment

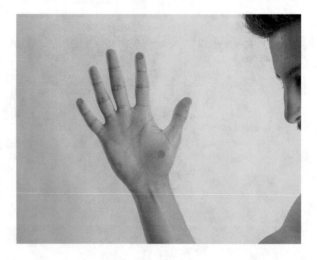

Fig. 5.31 Hand chart from the back demonstrates the site of radial nerve sensory assessment

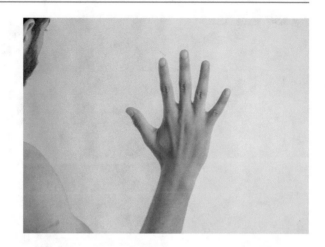

Fig. 5.32 OK sign for anterior interosseous nerve assessment

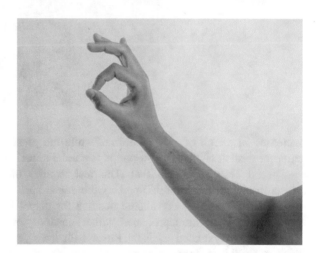

Fig. 5.33 Positive OK test if no resistance felt on trying to open the circle

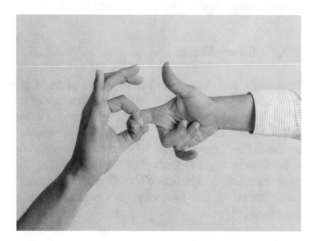

Fig. 5.34 Phalen test

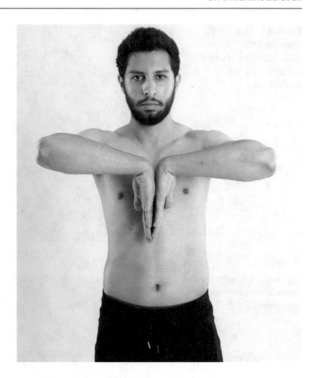

increases suspicion of PIN syndrome, while the presence of pain without wrist extensor weakness increases suspicion for radial tunnel syndrome [3, 10].

Special Tests: Phalen's Test. This test requires that the patient places their wrists in maximal flexion and presses the dorsal surfaces of their hands together (Fig. 5.34). The test is considered positive for carpal tunnel syndrome when the patient's symptoms are reproduced, with a sensitivity of 67.2% and a specificity of 92.9%. A closely related test is the Reverse Phalen's Test (Fig. 5.35), which is positive for carpal tunnel syndrome when placing the wrists in maximal extension while pressing the palms together reproduces symptoms [11–13].

5.2.1 Special Tests

Froment's Test. Ask the patient to grasp a piece of paper in the first web space on both sides while the caregiver holds the other side of the paper. A drawing or figure of the intended hand position should be provided to the patient and caregiver prior to conducting the test (Fig. 5.36). The test is considered positive if the patient is unable to hold onto the paper while the caregiver attempts to pull the paper away, or if the thumbs begin to flex rather than abduct (Fig. 5.37). A positive test suggests ulnar nerve injury. Maximal elbow flexion may require in case of query ulnar nerve involvement. If the symptoms exacerbate, cubital tunnel syndrome is more suggested [9].

Fig. 5.35 Reverse
Phalen test

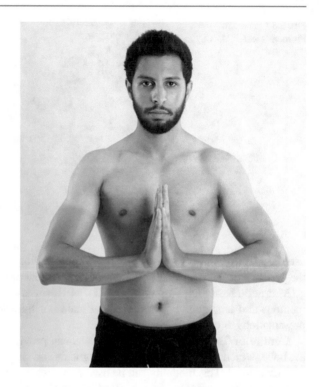

Fig. 5.36 Froment's test

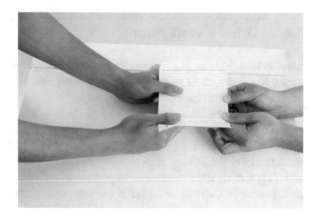

5.3   Radiology

Plain Film X-Ray (PXR). Standard PA, oblique, and lateral views of the wrist and
hand can be used to look for fractures, congenital deformities, arthritis, dysplasia,
and infections. The scaphoid view (wrist pronated, ulnar deviated, and in 30° supination) is useful for assessment of scaphoid fractures. The carpal tunnel view can be

Fig. 5.37 Positive Froment's test

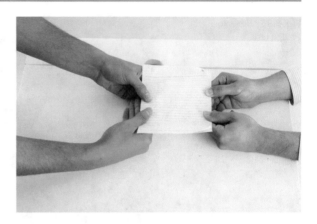

used to identify hook fractures. Finally, a stress radiograph may be obtained with the patient's hands in a clenched fist for the assessment of carpal instability [14, 15].

Magnetic Resonance Imaging (MRI). MRI is useful in the assessment of ligamentous and tendinous injuries, vascular status of the carpal bones, and delayed presentations of occult fractures.

Computer Tomography (CT). CT scans can provide more detailed images of the bone, which may be useful in both diagnosis and surgical planning.

Ultrasound. This modality can be used to assess tendon injuries.

Cineroentgenograph: It can be used to diagnose midcarpal instability [14].

5.4 Other Investigations

Conduction Studies. Nerve conduction velocity tests and electromyography can be useful in the diagnosis of nerve injuries as well as follow-up assessment of regeneration after treatment.

Laboratory Studies. A complete blood count (CBC), erythrocyte sedimentation rate (ESR), and C-reactive protein (CRP) are indicated in the case of suspected infection. In some cases, it may be important to assess for systemic diseases. The random blood glucose and HbA1C labs can test for diabetes mellitus. Serum T3, T4, and TSH can be used to identify hypothyroidism. Finally, anti-cyclic citrullinated proteins (anti-CCP) can be useful in the diagnosis of rheumatoid arthritis.

5.5 Algorithm for Hand Pain

Given the anatomical complexity of the hand and the broad range of potential pathologies, an algorithmic approach can be useful in working up a patient who presents with hand pain. For simplicity, pain of the wrist and hand can be classified into four etiologies: mechanical, neurologic, systemic, and psychologic.

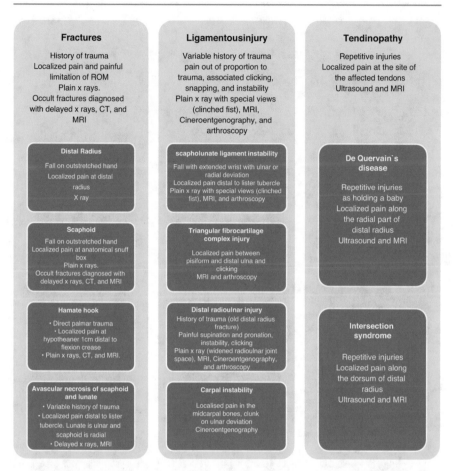

Fractures

History of trauma
Localized pain and painful
limitation of ROM
Plain x rays.
Occult fractures diagnosed
with delayed x rays, CT, and
MRI

Distal Radius

Fall on outstretched hand
Localized pain at distal
radius
X ray

Scaphoid

Fall on outstretched hand
Localized pain at anatomical snuff
box
Plain x rays.
Occult fractures diagnosed with
delayed x rays, CT, and MRI

Hamate hook

• Direct palmar trauma
• Localized pain at
hypotheaner 1cm distal to
flexion crease
• Plain x rays, CT, and MRI.

**Avascular necrosis of scaphoid
and lunate**

• Variable history of trauma
• Localized pain distal to lister
tubercle. Lunate is ulnar and
scaphoid is radial
• Delayed x rays, MRI

Ligamentousinjury

Variable history of trauma
pain out of proportion to
trauma, associated clicking,
snapping, and instability
Plain x ray with special views
(clinched fist), MRI,
Cineroentgenography, and
arthroscopy

scapholunate ligament instability

Fall with extended wrist with ulnar or
radial deviation
Localized pain distal to lister tubercle
Plain x ray with special views (clinched
fist), MRI, and arthroscopy

**Triangular fibrocartilage
complex injury**

Localized pain between
pisiform and distal ulna and
clicking
MRI and arthroscopy

Distal radioulnar injury

History of trauma (old distal radius
fracture)
Painful supination and pronation,
instability, clicking
Plain x ray (widened radioulnar joint
space), MRI, Cineroentgenography,
and arthroscopy

Carpal instability

Localised pain in the
midcarpal bones, clunk
on ulnar deviation
Cineroentgenography

Tendinopathy

Repetitive injuries
Localized pain at the site of
the affected tendons
Ultrasound and MRI

**De Quervain`s
disease**

Repetitive injuries
as holding a baby
Localized pain along
the radial part of
distal radius
Ultrasound and MRI

**Intersection
syndrome**

Repetitive injuries
Localized pain along
the dorsum of distal
radius
Ultrasound and MRI

Fig. 5.38 Chart shows an algorithm to sum up the causes of hand pain

Mechanical pain can be suspected when there is a history of trauma. Details of the traumatic mechanisms and subsequent signs and symptoms can be used to narrow the diagnosis (Fig. 5.38).

Any numbness or paresthesia suggests **neurologic pain**, and the distribution of pain can often help to narrow the initial diagnostic field (Fig. 5.39).

The **pain of systemic disease** can be suspected with any relevant positive findings in the general examination and past medical history. These include hematologic disease (e.g., leukemia, multiple myeloma), metabolic and endocrine conditions (e.g., acromegaly, diabetes mellitus, gout, pseudogout, hyperparathyroidism, Paget's disease, pregnancy), and rheumatologic disorders (e.g., psoriasis, rheumatoid arthritis, scleroderma, systemic lupus erythematosus).

Finally, **psychological pain** is a diagnosis of exclusion and should be suspected with positive psychological stressors, or when there are positive mood or affective symptoms upon examination.

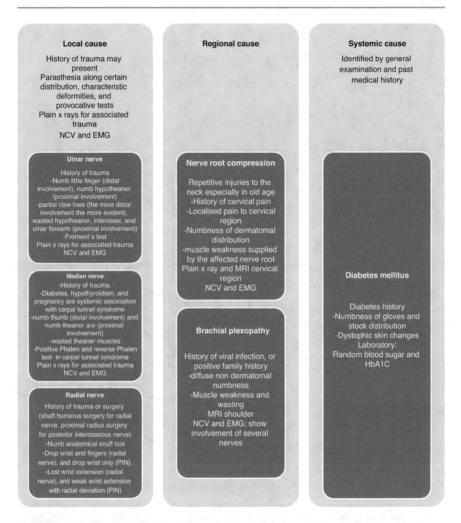

Fig. 5.39 Chart shows an algorithm to sum up the causes of neurologic hand pain

References

1. Dahaghin S, Bierma-Zeinstra SM, Reijman M, Pols HA, Hazes JM, Koes BW. Prevalence and determinants of one month hand pain and hand related disability in the elderly (Rotterdam study). Ann Rheum Dis. 2005;64(1):99–104.
2. Grice KO. The use of occupation-based assessments and intervention in the hand therapy setting—a survey. J Hand Ther. 2015;28(3):300–6.
3. Aulicino PL, DuPuy TE. Clinical examination of the hand. In: Rehabilitation of the hand: surgery and therapy, vol. 4. St Louis: Mosby; 1995. p. 53–75.
4. Ball C, Pratt AL, Nanchahal J. Optimal functional outcome measures for assessing treatment for Dupuytren's disease: a systematic review and recommendations for future practice. BMC Musculoskelet Disord. 2013;14:131.

5. Fowler JR, Hughes TB. Scaphoid fractures. Clin Sports Med. 2015;34:37–50.
6. Ağır I, Aytekin MN, Küçükdurmaz F, Gökhan S, Cavuş UY. Anatomical localization of Lister's tubercle and its clinical and surgical importance. Open Orthop J. 2014;8:74–7.
7. Rajan PV, Day CS. Scapholunate ligament insufficiency. J Hand Surg Am. 2015;40:583–5.
8. Johnsson PM, Eberhardt K. Hand deformities are important signs of disease severity in patients with early rheumatoid arthritis. Rheumatology. 2009;48(11):1398–401.
9. Tubiana R, Thomine JM, Mackin E. Examination of the hand and wrist. Boca Raton: CRC Press; 1998.
10. Collins S, Visscher P, De Vet HC, Zuurmond WW, Perez RS. Reliability of the Semmes Weinstein monofilaments to measure coetaneous sensibility in the feet of healthy subjects. Disabil Rehabil. 2010;32(24):2019–27.
11. Duckworth AD, Jenkins PJ, McEachan JE. Diagnosing carpal tunnel syndrome. J Hand Surg Am. 2014;39:1403–7.
12. LeBlanc KE, Cestia W. Carpal tunnel syndrome. Am Fam Physician. 2011;83:952–8.
13. Rayegani SM, Adybeik D, Kia MA. Sensitivity and specificity of two provocative tests (Phalen's test and Hoffmann-Tinel's sign) in the diagnosis of carpal tunnel syndrome. J Orthop Med. 2004;26(2):51–3.
14. Van Linthoudt D. Clinical presentation, imaging, and treatment of digital osteoarthritis. Rev Med Suisse. 2010;6(240):564–6568.
15. Hunter JM, Schneider LH, Mackin EJ, Callahan AD. Rehabilitation of the hand. Surgery and therapy. St. Louis: C. V. Mosby Company; 1990.

Pelvis, Hip, and Thigh

6

Mona Salah Mohamed Farhan, Viktor Krebs,
Ahmed K. Emara, and Nicolas S. Piuzzi

6.1 History

6.1.1 Personal History

Age of the patient and the onset of complaints can provide clue to the diagnosis. Deformity of progressive course in adolescence can suggest hip dysplasia while painful limitation of the hip in elderly obese can suggest primary osteoarthritis. The **level of residence** and he uses stairs or not can provide a clue to impact of pain on the activity level. Certain **occupation and sport activities** are at higher risk for hip disorders. History of heavy lifting can predispose to arthritis.

6.1.2 Present History

Pain: Analysis of pain can help reach the diagnosis [1].

M. S. M. Farhan
Orthopedic & Traumatology, Faculty of Medicine, Ain Shams University Hospital, Cairo, Egypt

Healthcare & Hospital Management, American University in Cairo AUC, Cairo, Egypt

Orthopedic & Traumatology, General Air Force Hospital, Cairo, Egypt

Medicine/Surgery "MBBCh", Faculty of Medicine, Ain Shams University, Cairo, Egypt

V. Krebs · A. K. Emara · N. S. Piuzzi (✉)
Department of Orthopedic Surgery, Cleveland Clinic Foundation, Cleveland, OH, USA
e-mail: piuzzin@ccf.org

- **Onset, course, and duration**: Sudden onset is more suggestive to mechanical factors.
- **Site, radiation, and character**: Hip pain is usually in groin and can referred anteriorly, medially, and laterally. Knee referral via obturator branch is not uncommon and can be the presenting pain. C sign may indicate an intra-articular hip pathology.
- **Intensity**: Quantify the intensity of the pain on a numerical scale from 1 to 10 can provide an idea about significance of pain.
- **Impact**: Another measure for the severity is the effect of this pain on the daily routine, work, and sleep.
- **What aggravates and what relieves**: Pain that increases with activities, and relieved by rest can suggest pain of arthritis. Pain due to tumor or infection origin may be constant and nocturnal.

Deformity (shortening and lengthening) and **limping**.

Stiffness: Especially in the morning may associate inflammatory etiology. It can be expressed in the form of difficult daily activities as putting on socks and going up stairs.

Affection of other joints: Associated rheumatoid hand may suggest rheumatoid arthritis etiology for the hip condition.

History of trauma may indicate the etiology of osteoarthritis.

Constitutional symptoms: Fever, nocturnal sweating, pain, and cachexia may indicate infection etiology as hip tuberculosis.

Mechanical symptoms: Clicking, snapping, catching, popping, and locking may indicate intra-articular loose body or labral tear [2].

Hip function can be objectively assessed using validated hip scores that can be used in the initial visit and in the follow-up visits especially after treatment. Among them, Harris Scoring System and WOMAC hip scores are commonly used [2].

6.1.3 Past History

Medications: Steroid intake history can suggest the development of avascular necrosis hip and to be the cause of symptoms.

Surgical history: provide insight regarding the previous scars and the possible difficulties that are anticipated in the future surgeries if needed.

Medical history: History of certain diseases as rheumatoid arthritis, tuberculosis is important to outline the possible diagnosis.

6.2 Clinical Examination

6.2.1 Inspection

Exposure by undressing to underwear as possible is required to inspect the whole lower limb.

Fig. 6.1 Inspect from the front for skin scars, sinuses, discoloration, swellings, muscle wasting (e.g., secondary to infection, disuse, polio) and deformity

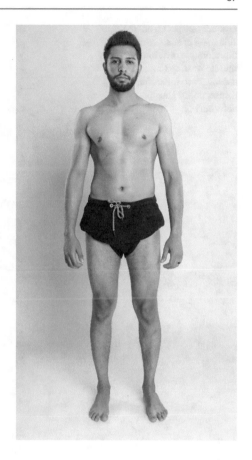

Inspect from the front (Fig. 6.1), sides (Fig. 6.2), and back (Fig. 6.3) for skin **scars**, **sinuses**, **discoloration**, **swellings**, and muscle **wasting** (e.g., secondary to infection, disuse, polio). Inspect for any **deformity** in the sagittal plane (increased lumbar lordosis suggestive of fixed flexion deformity of the hip) and in the coronal view searching for scoliosis (whether primary or compensatory to hip adduction or abduction deformity), pelvic tilt (may be due to scoliosis, apparent shortening, or true shortening), knee, or foot deformities [1, 2].

Observe the **gait** from the front, sides, and behind. Try to assess stride length, its components, and the possible associated stiffness, shortening (short limb gait), pain (antalgic gait) and gluteal insufficiency (Trendelenburg gait).

Patient with **limb length discrepancy** can be suspected by compensated plantarflexion of the foot on the short side, or by flexion of the knee on the other side. Most frequently, the discrepancy is countered by pelvic tilting. The latter may in turn be compensated by the development of a lumbar scoliosis. Suspected cases are asked to stand on book blocks of equal height with previous known height until leveling of the pelvis and patient's feeling of the leveling [2].

Fig. 6.2 Inspect from the side for skin scars, sinuses, discoloration, swellings, muscle wasting (e.g., secondary to infection, disuse, polio) and deformity

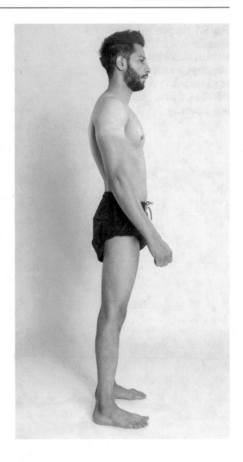

Trendelenburg test is performed by asking the patient to look at a wall without supporting by his/her hands and to elevate each limb and looking for possible sagging of the sound side to interpret the test as positive (Figs. 6.4 and 6.5).

6.2.2 Palpation

It cannot be assessed by telemedicine. However, the patient is instructed to draw the possible sites of pain using black marker. This may be of help to determine the tender points as a substitute to the palpation. Another method is to provide the patient with a drawing chart containing the required site of compression to elicit tenderness.

Fig. 6.3 Inspect from the
back for skin scars,
sinuses, discoloration,
swellings, muscle wasting
(e.g., secondary to
infection, disuse, polio)
and deformity

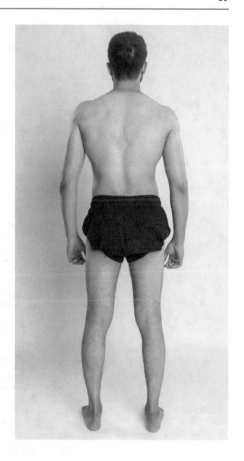

6.2.3 Range of Motion

The use of well-designed software in telemedicine can accurately assess the range
of motion and save the data precisely for follow-up comparison and research conduct. Active range of motion can be performed via telemedicine [3, 4].

Flexion: Ask the patient to lie supine, then flex each hip once a time as possible
(Fig. 6.6). An angle between the thigh and horizontal line is the degree of flexion.

Normal range of hip flexion is from 0° to 130°.

Extension: Ask the patient to lie supine at the couch edge. Then, ask him/her to
lie down one limb a time (Fig. 6.7). An angle between the thigh and horizontal line
is the degree of extension.

Normal range of hip extension is from 0° to 25° [2, 3].

Abduction and adduction: putting the camera at a higher level. So, looking
from the top view. Ask the patient to lie supine then move the thighs away from each
other as possible (Fig. 6.8), then each limb toward the other side (overcrossing) as
possible (Fig. 6.9). The degree of adduction and abduction is measured by calculating an angle between the thigh and vertical line passing through the middle of torso.

Fig. 6.4 Trendelenburg test

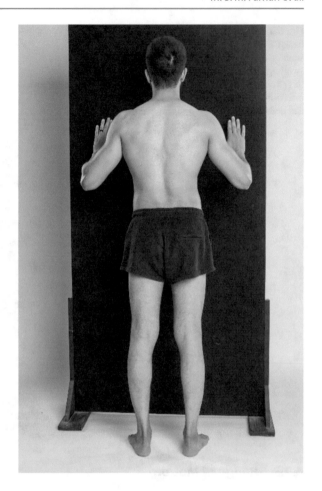

Normal range for hip abduction, from 0° to 45°. While normal degree for hip adduction, from 0° to 25° [2].

Internal and external rotation: Ask the patient to sit on couch edge. Then to move the legs away from each other as possible (Fig. 6.10) then each limb toward the other side (overcrossing) as possible (Fig. 6.11). The degree of internal rotation and external rotation is measured by calculating an angle between the leg and vertical line passing through the knee.

Normal range for hip internal rotation, from 0° to 25°. While normal range for hip external rotation, from 0° to 45° [2, 3].

Fixed flexion deformities: An alternative to Thomas test that can be conducted via telemedicine is to ask the patient to lie supine then to start in knee chest position (Fig. 6.12) and ask to extend each limb actively (Fig. 6.13). The angle between the thigh and horizontal line of the couch is the degree of fixed flexion deformity [3, 4].

Fig. 6.5 Trendelenburg test, looking for possible sagging, to interpret the result

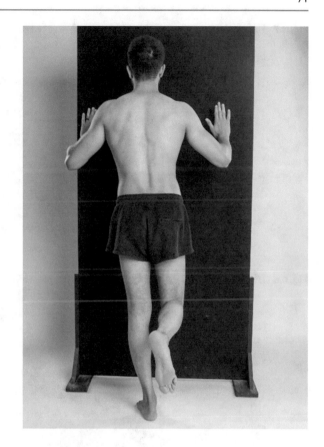

Fig. 6.6 Hip flexion

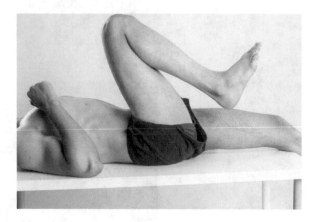

Fig. 6.7 Hip extension

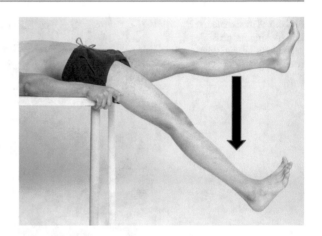

Fig. 6.8 Hip abduction

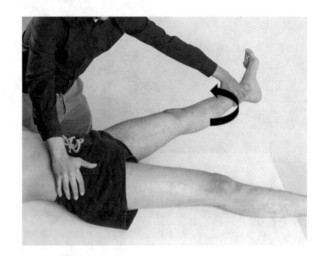

Fig. 6.9 Hip adduction

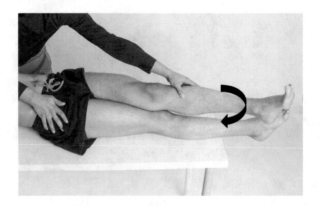

Fig. 6.10 Hip internal rotation

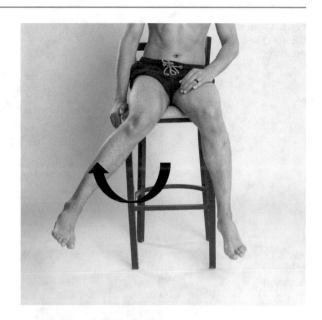

Fig. 6.11 Hip external rotation

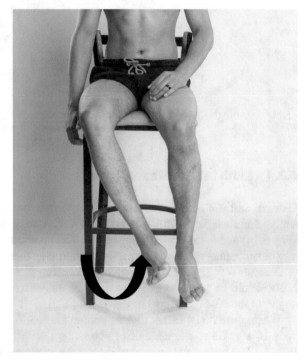

Fig. 6.12 Fixed flexion
deformity test, knee chest
position

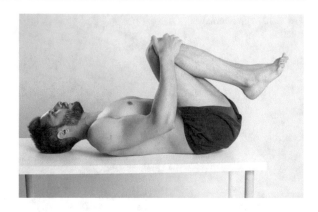

Fig. 6.13 Fixed flexion
deformity test, active leg
extension

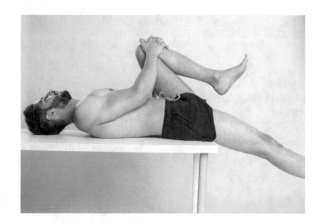

6.2.4   Limb Length Measurements

Galeazzi test can be effectively conducted via telemedicine. Ask the patient to lie supine and then flex both knees and hips 45°. A static shot is taken from the top (Fig. 6.14) and the side views (Fig. 6.15). The interpretation of hip and knee etiology of shortening can easily be performed utilizing these two static images.

Another way to know limb length discrepancy is that in the normal patient the heels should be level, and the plane of the anterior superior iliac spines at right angles to the edge of the couch (Fig. 6.16) [2, 3].

Where there is significant true shortening the heels will not be level (the discrepancy is a guide to the amount of shortening) and the pelvis will not be tilted (Fig. 6.17). The site and amount of shortening must now be further investigated.

However, as we cannot measure the degree of limb length discrepancy or conduct the tests identifying the site of shortening, we recommend relying on CT scanogram to accurately determine the degree of shortening as well as the site of shortening.

Fig. 6.14 Galeazzi test to assess limb length discrepancy, top view

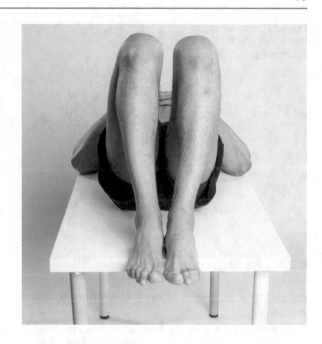

Fig. 6.15 Galeazzi test to assess limb length discrepancy, side view

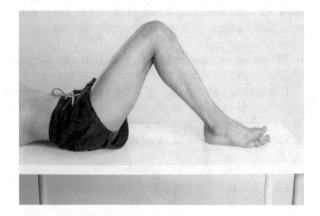

Fig. 6.16 Another way to assess limb length discrepancy

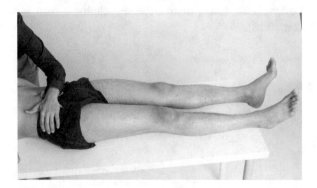

Fig. 6.17 Another way to assess limb length discrepancy

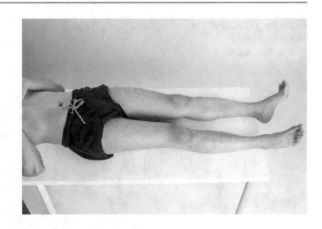

6.2.5 Radiographic Evaluation

Imaging will be used judiciously to confirm the diagnosis in telemedicine. These may include:

X-rays: Pelvis showing both hips, A-P, and lateral hip views, to look for fractures, arthritis, dysplasia, AVN, and infections. Moreover, plain X-ray lumbosacral spine AP and lateral may be asked in case of doubt as regard the possible source of pain. Scanograms can be used to measure the limb length discrepancy and to determine its components.

Magnetic resonance imaging (MRI): can diagnose hidden stress fractures, early stages of AVN.

Computed tomography (CT) scans: to see detailed images of bones of the pelvis and to plain the surgery as in dysplastic cases. CT scanogram can measure limb length discrepancy even in presence of deformities.

Ultrasound: can be of value in case of suspected septic arthritis [5].

6.2.6 Algorithm for Hip Pain Assessment

A mind map can be followed to reach the diagnosis. For simplicity, pain of hip can be insidious, acute, or overuse. Psychologic pain is the diagnosis of exclusion (Fig. 6.18).

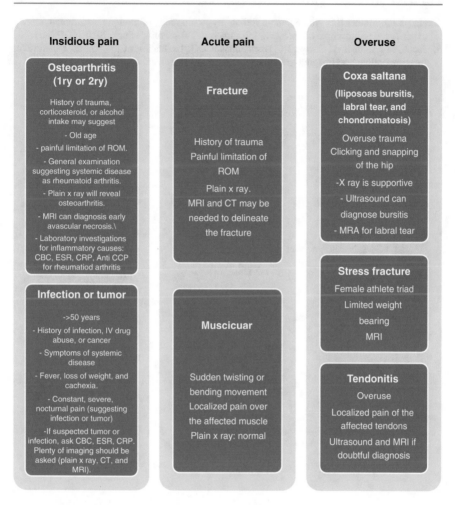

Fig. 6.18 Chart shows an algorithm for hip pain assessment

References

1. DeAngelis NA, Busconi BD. Assessment and differential diagnosis of the painful hip. Clin Orthop Relat Res. 2003;406(1):11–8.
2. McRae R. Clinical orthopaedic examination. London: Churchill Livingstone/Elsevier; 2010.
3. Ponte SM, Souza LM, da Costa BC, et al. Comparative analysis of neural mobilization and rhythmic stabilization in range of motion and hip pain. Manual therapy. Posturol Rehabil J 2019;17:17–9.

4. Harris JD, Mather RC, Nho SJ, et al. Reliability of hip range of motion measurement among experienced arthroscopic hip preservation surgeons. J Hip Preserv Surg. 2020;7(1):77–84.
5. Jacobson JA, Bedi A, Sekiya JK, Blankenbaker DG. Evaluation of the painful athletic hip: imaging options and imaging-guided injections. Am J Roentgenol. 2012;199(3):516–24.

Knee

7

Mahmoud Ahmed Elshobaky, Michael Erossy,
Carlos Higuera, and Jonathan Schaffer

7.1   History Taking

Age. Acute knee injuries, especially ligamentous and meniscal lesions, are especially common in young athletes. On the other hand, degenerative changes are more common in elderly patients, and may progress to osteoarthritis [1].

Mechanism of Injury. Following a traumatic event, it is very important to ask the patient about the detailed sequence of events leading to the injury. While contact injuries are often associated with fractures, non-contact twisting injuries are often associated with ligamentous injuries [1].

Pain. The specific characteristics of a patient's knee pain provide important diagnostic value. Pain on the medial aspect of the knee can suggest medial compartment arthritis, *genu varum*, pes anserinus tendinitis, or a medial meniscal lesion. Lateral knee pain, on the other hand, can be associated with lateral meniscal pathology or iliotibial tract syndrome. Anterior knee pain is one of the most common complaints in the orthopedic clinic, and the differential diagnosis includes quadriceps weakness, patellofemoral arthritis, osteochondritis dissecans (OCD) of the patella, pigmented villonodular synovitis (PVNS), and quadriceps or patellar tendinitis. The onset can also be diagnostically important, with an insidious onset and progressive course suggesting degenerative lesions like osteoarthritis and an acute onset suggestive of a traumatic etiology. The intensity of the pain can assist with diagnosis and evaluation, and it may be useful to ask the patient to rate pain on a numerical 1–10

M. A. Elshobaky (✉)
Orthopedic & Traumatology, Faculty of Medicine, Ain Shams University Hospital,
Cairo, Egypt

Medicine/Surgery "MBBCh", Faculty of Medicine, Ain Shams University, Cairo, Egypt

M. Erossy · C. Higuera · J. Schaffer
Department of Orthopedic Surgery, Cleveland Clinic Foundation, Cleveland, OH, USA

K. M. Emara, N. S. Piuzzi (eds.), *The Principles of Virtual Orthopedic Assessment*,
https://doi.org/10.1007/978-3-030-80402-2_7

point-scale. Pain that is aggravated by activities and relieved by rest can suggest arthritis, whereas pain associated with a tumor or infection is more commonly constant and nocturnal [2].

Stiffness. A limited range of motion with associated pain is most commonly caused by inflammation, and suggestive of synovitis. Other causes of stiffness include a history of fracture with delayed rehabilitation, quadriceps contractures, patella baja, and osteoarthritis [2].

Instability. In a young patient with a history of a non-contact injury, it is important to differentiate between a ligamentous injury and patellofemoral pain which can cause quadriceps inhibition. Whereas the former is typically painless and occurs with pivoting movement, the latter is more commonly associated with pain when walking upstairs or with any movement that increases stress on the patellofemoral joint. Consequently, it is very important to ask the patient about the frequency of giving away, the circumstances under which this occurs, and whether there is pain [1, 2].

Past Medical History. The patient's history can be an important factor in contextualizing their clinical presentation and making appropriate risk assessments. Patients with a history of rheumatoid arthritis may exhibit a valgus deformity. Patients with a history of osteoarthritis, on the other hand, may exhibit a varus deformity. A history of autoimmune disease treated with cortisone medication can increase the risk of osteonecrosis. Prior fractures of the tibial plateau or the patella can also cause deformity and accelerate arthritis [1, 2].

7.2   Examination

Inspection. The examination can begin with a visual inspection of the knees, from the anterior, lateral, and posterior views (Figs. 7.1, 7.2, and 7.3). Careful inspection can reveal any swelling, muscle wasting, or scars from previous injuries or

Fig. 7.1 Inspection of the knee from the front

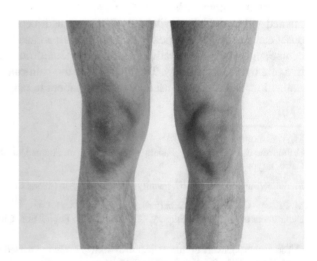

Fig. 7.2 Inspection of the
knee from sides

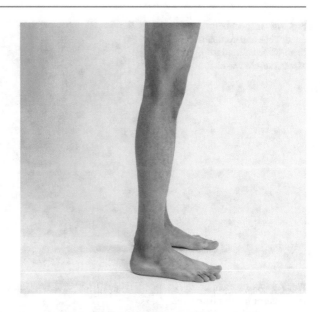

Fig. 7.3 Inspection of the
knee from the back

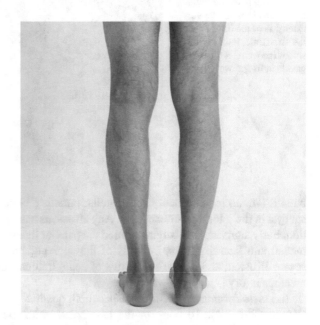

operations. When **swelling** is present, note whether the swelling is confined to the
limits of the synovial cavity and suprapatellar pouch. Swelling limited by these
anatomical boundaries can suggest effusion, hemarthrosis, pyarthrosis, or a space-
occupying lesion in the joint. If the swelling extends beyond the joint cavity, infection (of the joint, femur, or tibia), tumor, or injury should be suspected. Any **lumps**
or localized swelling should be noted as well, as these can suggest prepatellar

Fig. 7.4 Inspect both quadriceps and compare them while relaxed to assess muscle wasting

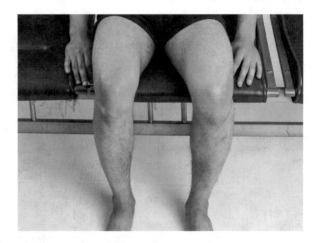

Fig. 7.5 Assessment of the extensor mechanism: ask the patient to straighten the leg and look for active extension of the limb. At the same time, look for the smooth movement of the patella in its groove

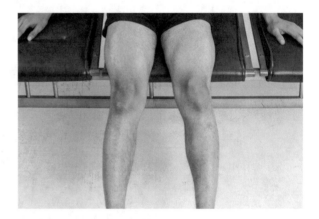

bursitis ("housemaid's knee"), infrapatellar bursitis ("clergyman's knee"), a meniscal cyst in the joint line, or exostosis. Any **effusions** can also be detected on inspection. Early signs include bulging around the patellar ligament and obliteration of the medial and lateral gutters. Fullness of the suprapatellar pouch indicates a more severe effusion, and can be suggestive of acute trauma, such as a fracture or ligamentous injury [2].

To assess for muscle **wasting**, inspect both quadriceps and compare them while relaxed (Fig. 7.4). To perform the assessment with the quadriceps contracted, instruct the patient to place a towel underneath their popliteal fossa and push against it [2].

Extensor mechanism: With the patient sitting with his legs over the end of the examination couch, ask him to straighten the leg and look for active extension of the limb (Fig. 7.5). You can ask the patient to do straight leg raise also to assess integrity of extensor mechanism [1, 2] (Fig. 7.6).

Fig. 7.6 Another method to assess the extensor mechanism: ask the patient to do straight leg raise also to assess integrity of extensor mechanism

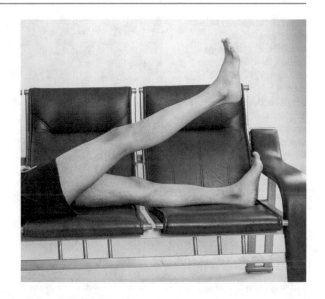

To assess the **patella**, a lateral view of the standing patient can reveal genu recurvatum. The position of the patella relative to the femoral condyles should also be observed in this position, as a high patella (*patella alta*) predisposes the patient to recurrent lateral dislocation (Fig. 7.2). From the anterior view of the standing patient, genu valgum may be noted. This is also a risk factor for recurrent patellar dislocation, especially as the Q angle increases and more lateral translational stress is placed upon the knee (Fig. 7.1). For further assessment of the patella, the patient should be asked to move to a seated position with knees flexed and hanging over the end of a couch or chair. Any torsional deformities of the femur or tibia may be observed from this view. In addition, if the patella is laterally displaced, the patient will be predisposed to instability, e.g., recurrent dislocation, or chondromalacia patellae. Next, ask the patient to extend their knees while watching the movement of their patella, which should move smoothly in the patellar groove. Any gross disturbance in patellar tracking should be noted [2] (Figs. 7.4 and 7.5).

Palpation. The sites of **tenderness** to palpation can provide diagnostic value. To assess for tenderness, the patient can be provided an image of the knee with regions for the patient to self-palpate (Fig. 7.7). The patient can also easily detect **temperature** during palpation and should be asked to report the location and extent of any heat and compare left and right sides. Increased heat can be indicative of rheumatoid arthritis, infection, rapidly growing tumors, or an inflammatory response to injury.

Range of Motion. Active ROM of the knee can be tested by asking the patient to place the camera in a lateral view and then extend and flex their knees (Figs. 7.8 and 7.9). While assessing for the ROM, any pain during the movement should be noted as well. If the patient cannot extend their knees actively, they likely may have an extension lag or a knee flexion deformity. To differentiate between these two etiologies, the patient can place the contralateral leg on the knee being examined. If doing

Fig. 7.7 Palpation map of the knee. 1: vastus medialis, 2: quadriceps tendon, 3: iliotibial band and vastus lateralis, 4: medial joint line and medial collateral ligament, 5: patella, 6: patellar tendon, 7: lateral joint line and lateral collateral ligament, 8: pes anserinus, 9: tibial tuberosity, 10: fibula head and tibialis anterior

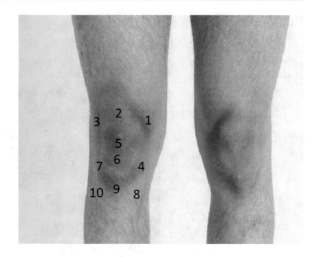

Fig. 7.8 Full active knee flexion

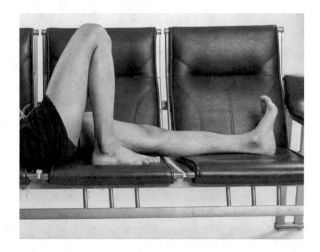

so increases the extension range, then the limited ROM is likely due to quadriceps weakness. If the extension range does not increase, then a knee flexion deformity is more likely (Fig. 7.10). This differentiation can also be made with the assistance of a caregiver if by asking the caregiver to apply downward force on the knee, a similar assessment can be made [1, 2] (Fig. 7.11).

7.2.1 Special Tests

Gravity Test. This is a test for assessment of the posterior cruciate ligament (PCL). Rupture, detachment, or stretching of the PCL can result in posterior subluxation of the tibia, which can visually manifest as a striking deformity. To conduct the test,

Fig. 7.9 Full active knee extension

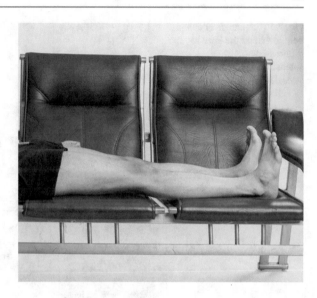

Fig. 7.10 Patient can place the contralateral leg on the knee being examined to differentiate between extension lag and flexion knee deformity

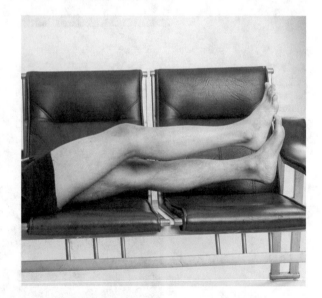

the knee should be flexed to 90° . The test is considered positive if a deformity is present (Fig. 7.12). An alternative method to assess PCL damage, ask the patient to lift their heel from the couch with their knee in 20° flexion. The test is considered positive if any posterior subluxation occurs [1] (Fig. 7.13).

Thessaly Test. This is a test for meniscal injury and is performed with the patient standing with their knees in 5° and 10° of flexion. The patient will then stand on one leg at a time, beginning with the unaffected side to gain familiarity and confidence with the movement. The patient can use a wall or other nearby fixed object to assist

Fig. 7.11 A caregiver can help to extend the knee to differentiate between extension lag and flexion knee deformity

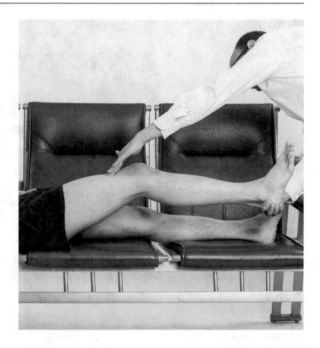

Fig. 7.12 Gravity test: PCL assessment: inspection of deformity (posterior subluxation) in patients with affected PCL with 90° flexed knee

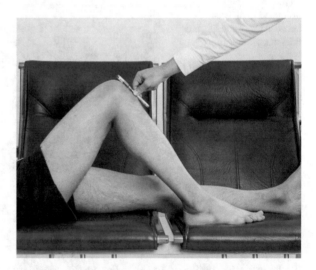

with balance while standing on one leg. The patient will then rotate slowly from side to side. The maneuver should be performed three times, and the test is considered positive if the patient experiences any joint line pain or sensations of locking or catching within the knee [1] (Figs. 7.14 and 7.15).

Special Note on Peroneal Injuries. Peroneal injuries are common complications in cases of suspected lateral collateral ligament injury and knee dislocation. Assessment of the peroneal nerve can be readily performed by observing the patient's ability to dorsiflex their ankle and big toe when asked to do so.

Fig. 7.13 PCL assessment: ask the patient to lift their heel from the couch with their knee in 20° flexion. The test is considered positive if any posterior subluxation

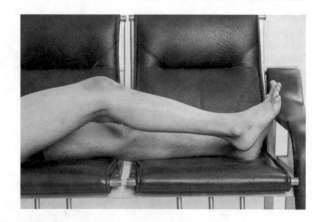

Fig. 7.14 Thessaly test (a): patient will stand on one leg at a time then rotate slowly from side to side. The maneuver should be performed three times, and the test is considered positive if the patient experiences pain, locking or catching

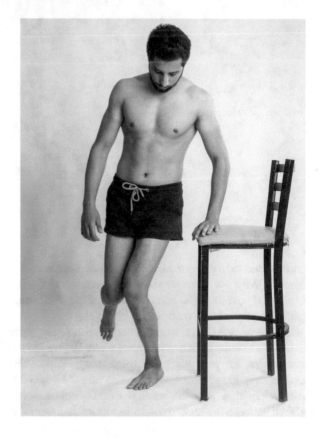

7.3   Radiology

Plain X-Ray (PXR). A set of X-rays should be ordered in the AP, lateral, and sky-line views. These allow for assessment of joint space narrowing as well as the pro-gression of osteoarthritis. Segond fracture, which is an avulsion of the anterolateral

Fig. 7.15 Thessaly test (b): patient will stand on one leg at a time then rotate slowly from side to side. The maneuver should be performed three times, and the test is considered positive if the patient experiences pain, locking or catching

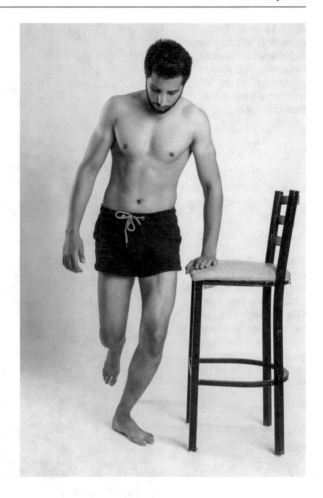

capsule secondary to an ACL tear, can be seen on an AP view if it is present. A standing AP view can also allow for assessment of any varus or valgus deformity. Other diagnoses such as bony avulsion of the tibial spine, fibular head avulsion, or MCL avulsion can be made using PXR [3].

In assessing **ACL function**, anterior subluxation of the tibia while the knee is in extension may be apparent in lateral view. To provide a more detailed radiographic assessment, the patient's lower thigh can be supported by a sandbag while they extend their leg against the resistance of a 7-kg weight. The limb should be in a neutral position with the patella pointing upwards, and the X-ray film cassette placed between the legs. To perform a more quantitative assessment, draw two lines parallel to the posterior cortex of the tibia, tangential to the medial tibial plateau and the medial femoral condyle. The distance between the two lines can then be measured, and is normally 3.5 mm ± 2 mm. A measurement of 10.2 mm ± 2.7 mm has a high diagnostic reliability for ACL tear, although the length may also be increased in the setting of a torn medial meniscus [4].

To assess **PCL function**, a sandbag can be placed behind the thigh and the proximal tibia can be pressed forcibly backwards with an approximate force of a 25-kg weight. This is repeated, and after the second preloading cycle, radiographs are taken while the same force is maintained.

The gap between the medial femoral and tibial condyles is measured, along with the distance between the lateral condyles. A displacement of approximately 8 mm on each side is indicative of an uncomplicated PCL tear. Excessive movement on the lateral or medial sides indicates posterolateral or posteromedial instability [4].

To assess for **varus and valgus instability**, stress valgus and varus views can be used. Comparing joint opening grades in neutral and stress views can allow for assessment of MCL, LCL, and PLC injury [3, 4].

Computed Tomography (CT). This modality is especially useful in the assessment of mechanical axis deviation, which can be accomplished using coronal malalignment measurements. CT may also be used to measure tibial tuberosity-trochlear groove (TT-TG) distance in cases of recurrent patellar dislocation to assess for femoral anteversion [5].

Magnetic Resonance Imaging (MRI). MRI is the gold standard in assessment of knee ligamentous and meniscal injuries. It allows an accurate assessment of the state of the cruciate and collateral ligaments in 80% of cases [6].

This flowchart explains how to approach knee assessment via telemedicine (Fig. 7.16).

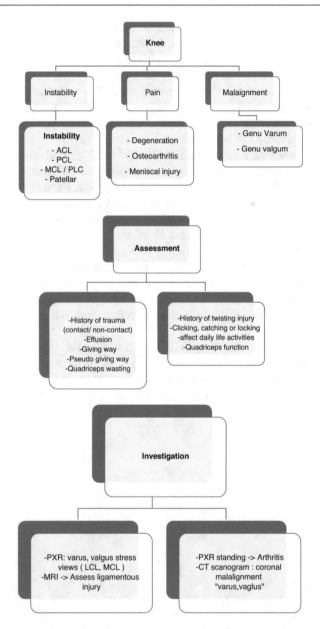

Fig. 7.16 Charts demonstrate how to approach knee assessment via telemedicine

References

1. McRae R. Clinical orthopaedic examination. London: Churchill Livingstone/Elsevier; 2010.
2. Bronstein RD, Schaffer JC. Physical examination of knee ligament injuries. J Am Acad Orthop Surg. 2017;25(4):280–7.
3. Toivanen AT, Arokoski JP, Manninen PS, Heliövaara M, Haara MM, Tyrväinen E, Niemitukia L, Kröger H. Agreement between clinical and radiological methods of diagnosing knee osteoarthritis. Scand J Rheumatol. 2007;36(1):58–63.
4. LaPrade RF, Heikes C, Bakker AJ, Jakobsen RB. The reproducibility and repeatability of varus stress radiographs in the assessment of isolated fibular collateral ligament and grade-III posterolateral knee injuries: an in vitro biomechanical study. JBJS. 2008;90(10):2069–76.
5. Beldame J, Bertiaux S, Roussignol X, Lefebvre B, Adam JM, Mouilhade F, Dujardin F. Laxity measurements using stress radiography to assess anterior cruciate ligament tears. Orthop Traumatol Surg Res. 2011;97(1):34–43.
6. Lee YS, Han SH, Jo J, Kwak KS, Nha KW, Kim JH. Comparison of 5 different methods for measuring stress radiographs to improve reproducibility during the evaluation of knee instability. Am J Sports Med. 2011;39(6):1275–81.

Lower Leg, Foot, and Ankle

8

Mohamed Amr Hemida, Stephen Pinney,
and Sara Lyn Miniaci-Coxhead

8.1   Overview

The ankle and foot are unique in their ability to bear and transmit an individual's total body weight. Any imbalance between the anatomical components of the foot and ankle can interfere with a patient's ability to walk, run, or even stand upright. Assessment of the ankle joint should always be done with an assessment of the ipsilateral foot and knee. The foot and ankle are anatomically complex, with 28 bones and 57 articulations. Understanding of the complex anatomy is important in assessment and diagnosis of foot and ankle problems [1].

The ankle joint is formed by three bones: the tibial plafond through the medial malleolus of the tibia, the distal end of the fibula, and the talus. The primary motion of the ankle joint is plantarflexion and dorsiflexion, although it also plays a secondary role in inversion, eversion, and rotation. Medially, the joint is supported by two ligaments: the deltoid ligament and the calcaneonavicular ligament. Laterally, it is supported by four ligaments: the anterior talofibular ligament (ATFL), posterior talofibular ligament (PTFL), calcaneal fibular ligament (CFL), and the lateral talocalcaneal ligament (LTCL) [1]. The distal fibula and the distal tibia are connected by a syndesmosis consisting of several ligaments: anterior inferior tibiofibular ligament (AITFL), posterior inferior tibiofibular ligament (PITFL), transverse tibiofibular ligament (TTFL), and interosseous ligament (IOL) [2].

The foot can be anatomically divided into the hindfoot, midfoot, and forefoot. The hindfoot includes the subtalar joint, an articulation between the talus and the calcaneus responsible for inversion and eversion, the talonavicular joint, and the

M. A. Hemida
Orthopedic Surgery, Ain Shams University, Cairo, Egypt

S. Pinney (✉) · S. L. Miniaci-Coxhead
Department of Orthopedic Surgery, Cleveland Clinic Foundation, Cleveland, OH, USA
e-mail: pinneys5@ccf.org

© The Author(s), under exclusive license to Springer Nature Switzerland AG 2022
K. M. Emara, N. S. Piuzzi (eds.), *The Principles of Virtual Orthopedic Assessment*,
https://doi.org/10.1007/978-3-030-80402-2_8

calcaneocuboid joint. The midfoot includes the naviculocuneiform joint, the inter-cuneiform joints, and the tarsometatarsal joints (*Lisfranc joint*). The forefoot is comprised of 5 metatarsals and 14 phalanges which form metatarsophalangeal (MTP) joints, proximal interphalangeal (PIP) joints, and distal interphalangeal (DIP) joints. Each toe is comprised of three phalanges, except for the big toe, which is comprised of only two. All of these structures within the foot and ankle are sur-rounded by a network of vessels and nerves providing motor innervation, sensory innervation, and blood supply to the tissues [1, 2].

8.2 History

Age and **Sex**. Many diseases and fracture types are more prevalent in different age groups or among patients of a particular sex. Freiberg's disease, for example, is common in female patients 13–18 years old [3].

Activities. Different motions can predispose patients to different pathologies as well, so it is important to ask about occupation, residence, and athletic activities. For example, flexor hallucis longus tendonitis is more common in dancers (espe-cially *on pointe*) and gymnasts. Other behaviors like smoking can also be risk fac-tors for various pathologies and are also important to explore when taking the patient's history [4].

Mechanism of Injury. If the patient's complaint is related to trauma, it is impor-tant to determine the exact mechanism of injury. Fall on an inverted ankle often results in fifth metatarsal base fracture, ATLF injury, or CFL injury. Trauma from an eversion mechanism is more commonly associated with deltoid ligament injury and syndesmotic injury. Hyper dorsiflexion, on the other hand, can result in Achilles tendon injury and talar fracture [4].

Past Medical and **Surgical History**. Many systemic conditions may manifest in the foot. A diabetic patient, for example, may develop diabetic Charcot ankle. Cardiac conditions like heart failure may cause a pitting edema in the foot and ankle. A history of traumatic brain injury may result in an acquired spastic equin-ovarus deformity [5].

Pain. Pain is the most common complaint in orthopedic foot and ankle patients. Determining the location of pain, type of pain, palliation, provocation, and its effects on patient activities such as walking can help narrow the differential diagnosis and determine the severity of the problem. Pain that wakes the patient from sleep may be due to a muscle spasm, as the protective mechanism preventing spasm is relaxed during sleep and can result in severe pain. Generalized pain is most often associated with degenerative changes, complex regional pain syndrome, or nerve injury. Localized pain that can be pointed to with a single finger may be more indicative of a bony fracture or ligamentous injury. Pain that increases with weight-bearing is usually indicative of arthritis, fracture, or ligament injury. If the pain is exacerbated by footwear, a deformity such as hallux valgus or bunion may be the cause of pain. If the pain increases when walking on uneven ground, the cause can often be attrib-uted to pathology of the subtalar joint or peroneal tendons. If there is an anterior impingement of the ankle, patients usually complain of pain while going up the stairs. Conversely, in the cause of posterior impingement, patients usually complain of pain while going down the stairs. The surgeon should also ask the patient about any pain in the spine, as spinal etiologies such as lumbar disc herniation may also present as pain in the foot and ankle [4, 5].

Stiffness. Stiffness, especially in the early morning, is often indicative of rheumatoid arthritis and can also suggest osteoarthritis. Post-traumatic fracture malunion can also cause stiffness [5].

Swelling. Swelling can be categorized as general or localized. There are many causes of generalized swelling including rheumatoid arthritis, septic arthritis, osteoarthritis, severe soft tissue injury, and systemic diseases like heart failure. Localized swelling of the medial ankle is often associated with deltoid ligament injury or a fracture of the medial malleolus. Localized swelling of the lateral ankle can be suggestive of a lateral malleolus fracture [4].

Examination

Inspection. To fully inspect the ankle and foot, the patient should be asked to remove their shoes and socks and expose their legs above the knee level. Inspection should be performed from the anterior (Fig. 8.1), lateral (Fig. 8.2), medial (Fig. 8.3), plantar (Fig. 8.4), and dorsal (Fig. 8.5) perspectives. Inspection should be done with the patient in the standing and seated position. Any deformities of alignment, scars, swelling, color changes, callouses, and ulcerations should be noted [6].

With the patient in a natural standing position and the camera in an anterior position (Fig. 8.6), the surgeon can make note of the degree of external rotation in the sagittal plane. The normal degree of rotation is 5–18°. Causes of increased external

Fig. 8.1 Inspection of the anterior aspect of the foot and ankle

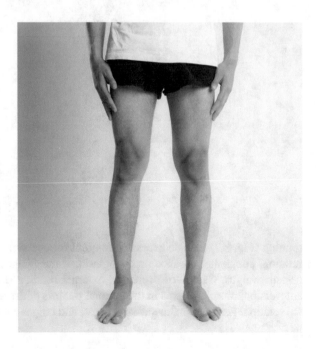

Fig. 8.2 Inspection of the lateral aspect of the foot and ankle

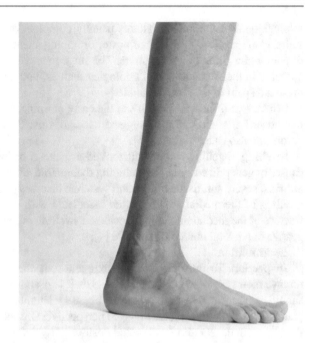

Fig. 8.3 Inspection of the medial aspect of the foot and ankle

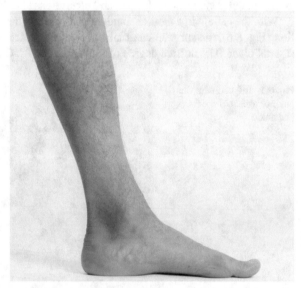

rotation (Fig. 8.7) include excessive femoral retroversion, excessive tibial external rotation, congenital absence or hypoplasia of the fibulae, pes valgus, and talipes calcaneovalgus. Causes of decreased external rotation (Fig. 8.8) include femoral anteversion, muscle spasms in the internal rotators of the hip, excessive tibial internal rotation, genu varum, metatarsus varus, and talipes equinovarus [5, 6].

Fig. 8.4 Inspection of the plantar aspect of the foot

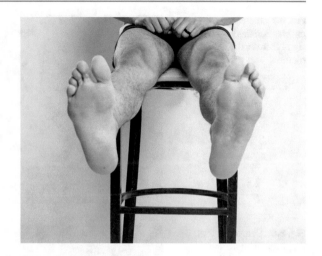

Fig. 8.5 Inspection of the dorsal aspect of the foot

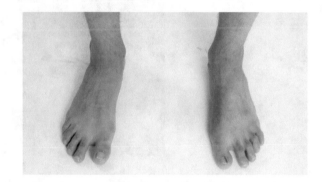

Fig. 8.6 Assessment of foot progression angle. Normal angle is 5–18° external rotation to the sagittal plane

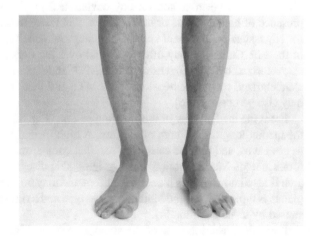

Fig. 8.7 Increased foot progression angle: toe out sign "Increased external rotation"

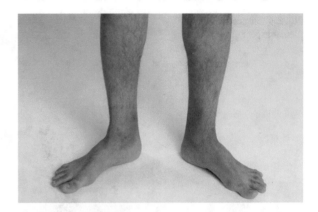

Fig. 8.8 Decreased foot progression angle: toe in sign

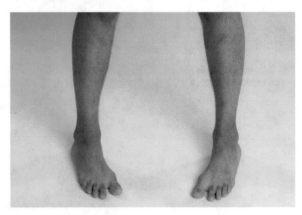

The alignment of toes should also be inspected from the standing position. The big toe should be inspected for any deviation from the midline to determine the presence of hallux valgus or hallux varus. The lesser toes should also be inspected for any issues in alignment such as hammer toe, which is characterized by flexion of the PIP. Callouses may often be found over the dorsum of the PIP. Mallet toe, characterized by hyperextension of the MTP and flexion of the DIP, and claw toe, characterized by hyperextension of the MTP and flexion of both the PIP and DIP, may also be observed [6].

From the medial view of the standing patient (Fig. 8.3), the surgeon can observe the medial longitudinal arch of the foot. A high medial longitudinal arch is known as pes cavus, and may be caused by residual compartment syndrome, residual club foot, Charcot–Marie–Tooth disease, or idiopathic disease. An abnormally collapsed arch is also known as pes planus or flat foot and may be caused by vertical talus. Pes planus is typically classified into a flexible type and a rigid type, which is frequently caused by tarsal coalition [4].

From the posterior view of the standing patient (Fig. 8.9), the hindfoot can be assessed. The valgus angle can be measured by tracing bilateral lines bisecting the heel and is normally 5–10°. An increased valgus angle is seen in cases of advanced

Fig. 8.9 Inspection of the posterior aspect of the foot and ankle

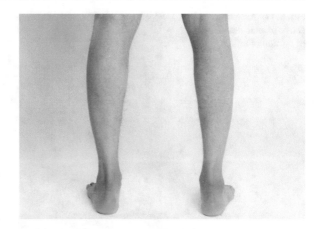

Fig. 8.10 Inspection of the gait: foot drop gait is evident

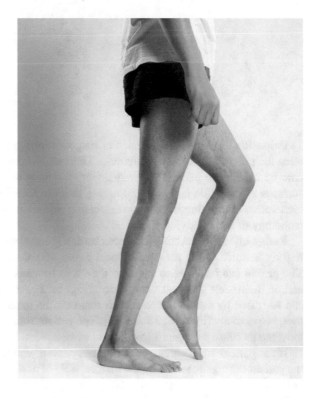

arthritis and Charcot arthropathy. Varus inclination, on the other hand, may be seen in malunited ankle fractures or be idiopathic.

Gait. Inspection of the gait from the anterior, posterior, and laterally from both sides may reveal abnormalities such as an antalgic gait which may be accompanied by painful conditions (Fig. 8.10) [5].

Fig. 8.11 Assessment of
active plantar flexion range
of motion of ankle

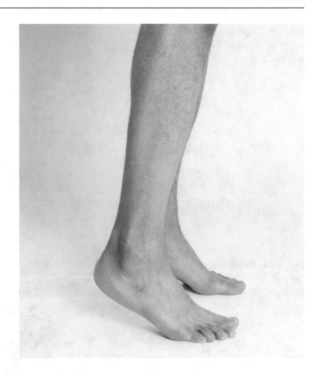

Palpation. The main importance of palpation of the foot and ankle is to determine the point of maximum tenderness. This can be accomplished in the telemedicine by asking the patient to use their index fingers to palpate varying sites and surfaces of the ankle and foot and asking them to identify the point of maximum tenderness. Identifying the anatomic location of maximal tenderness may point to pathology of an underlying structure.

Range of Motion. Active ROM can be easily translated to the telemedicine setting by instructing the patient to repeat maneuvers demonstrated by the surgeon. The patient can be asked to stand on their toes to assess plantarflexion (Fig. 8.11) and on their heels to assess dorsiflexion (Fig. 8.12). Active inversion and eversion can be tested by asking the patient to stand on the inner and outer borders of the foot, respectively (Figs. 8.13 and 8.14). The patient should be asked if any of these movements cause pain, and ROM should be compared bilaterally [6].

If the patient has a caregiver or another person who is physically present with the patient during the telemedicine visit capable of assisting, passive ROM maneuvers can be performed. Assessment of passive ankle dorsiflexion can be performed with the caregiver holding the heel in neutral with the one hand and using the other hand to grasp at the midfoot, invert, and dorsiflex the ankle (Fig. 8.15). Normal passive ankle dorsiflexion is 20°. Stiffness may be caused by an ankle fracture or a posterior compartment pathology such as a gastrocnemius or soleus contracture. To differentiate these two possible causes of a posterior structure contracture, passive dorsiflexion should be repeated with 90° of knee flexion (Fig. 8.16). If the

Fig. 8.12 Assessment of active dorsiflexion range of motion of ankle

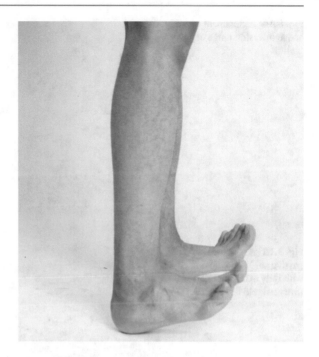

Fig. 8.13 Assessment of active eversion range of motion

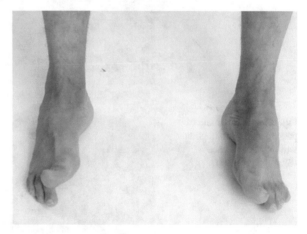

ROM does not change, the stiffness is due to soleus contracture. If the ROM improves with the knee in 90° of flexion, the stiffness is due to gastrocnemius contracture. Passive plantarflexion ROM can be assessed in a similar fashion (Fig. 8.17). Normal ROM is approximately 50°. To assess passive ROM of the first MTP joint, the caregiver can fix the head of the first metatarsal with their thumb and index finger, and use the other hand to manipulate the proximal phalanx of the big toe. Normal passive flexion and extension of the MTP joint are 40° and 60°, respectively (Fig. 8.18a, b) [5, 6].

Fig. 8.14 Assessment of
active inversion range of
motion

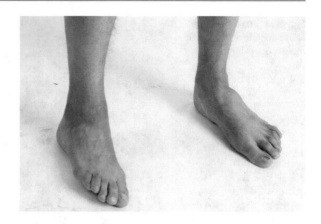

Fig. 8.15 Assessment of
passive ankle dorsiflexion
with fully extended knee
(Silfverskiold test)

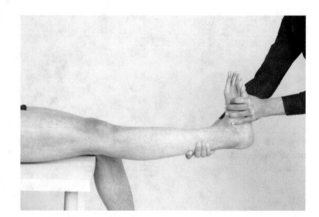

Fig. 8.16 Assessment of
passive ankle dorsiflexion
with 90° flexed knee
(Silfverskiold test)

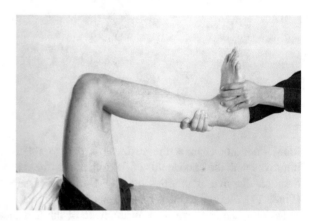

Fig. 8.17 Assessment of
ankle passive plantar
flexion

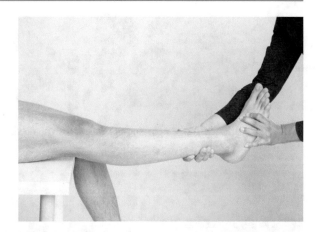

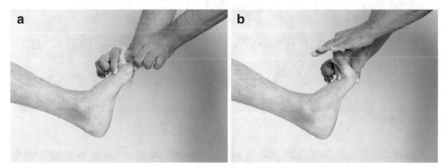

Fig. 8.18 (**a**, **b**) Assessment of passive range of motion of first metatarsophalangeal joint

8.2.1   Special Tests

Jack Test. This is a test to differentiate flexible from rigid flat foot. With the patient
in the standing position, the surgeon should observe the medial longitudinal arch.
The test is performed by having the caregiver dorsiflex the big toe. If arch reconstitution occurs, it is considered a flexible flat foot (Fig. 8.19a, b) [7].

Thompson's Test. This tests the integrity of the Achilles tendon. The patient is
asked to lie in the prone position with the feet hanging off the edge of the table. A
caregiver will need to squeeze the calf and repeat on the other leg for comparison.
If plantarflexion is lost on the affected side, the test is considered positive for an
Achilles tendon tear (Fig. 8.20a, b) [8].

Squeeze Test. To perform this test, a caregiver will need to squeeze the tibia and
fibular together at the midshaft. The test is positive for syndesmotic injury if this
motion elicits pain at the ankle.

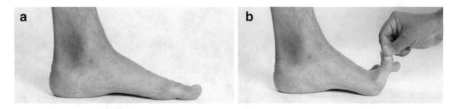

Fig. 8.19 (**a**, **b**) Jack Test: reconstitution of the arch with dorsiflexion of the big toe of standing patient

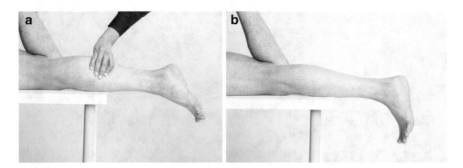

Fig. 8.20 (**a**, **b**) Thompson's test: intact tendon Achilles shows ankle plantar flexion with squeezing the calf

Coleman Block Test. The test is used to assess the flexibility of a cavovarus deformity of the hindfoot. This test is performed by placing the patient's foot on a wooden block that is 2.5–4 cm thick, with the heel and lateral border of the foot on the block while the first and third metatarsals are allowed to hang freely into plantarflexion and pronation. If the hindfoot deformity is corrected to neutral or valgus alignment, the deformity can be corrected with surgery of the forefoot. If the hindfoot deformity is not corrected by the wooden block, then a corrective hindfoot osteotomy will be needed to correct the deformity (Fig. 8.21) [4, 5].

Tip Toe Test. This test differentiates between a rigid and flexible pes planus deformity. In a flexible flat foot deformity, the medial longitudinal arch collapses upon weight-bearing but reconstitutes when the patient raises the foot onto their tiptoe (Fig. 8.22) [4].

8.3 Radiology

Plain Film X-Ray (PXR). PXR is usually indicated for the evaluation of fractures, loose bodies, and the presence of arthritis. AP and lateral views are standard and typically required, although special views such as the oblique and mortise views may be useful as well. A PXR with the foot rotated internally about 10° can be useful for assessing the syndesmosis. A syndesmotic injury is defined by increased tibiofibular clear space of more than 5.3 mm in AP view, tibiofibular overlap less

Fig. 8.21 Block test for assessment of hindfoot flexibility in cavovarus foot deformity

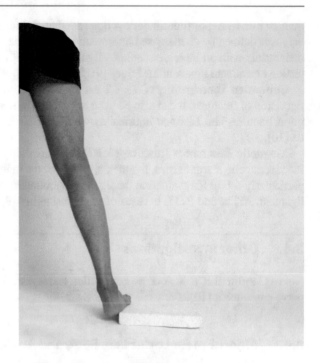

Fig. 8.22 Tip Toe test for assessment of pes planus deformity

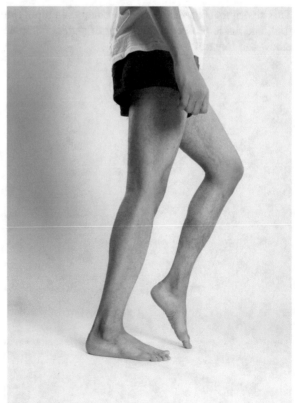

than 10 mm in AP, or tibiofibular overlap less than 2.8 mm in mortise view. Hallux valgus is defined by an increased intermetatarsal angle between the first and second metatarsals with an increased hallux valgus angle. PXR can also be used in stress testing to evaluate ligamentous injury [9].

Computed Tomography (CT). CT can be used to show further detail and configuration of fractures. It can also be used to evaluate intraarticular fractures such as pilon fractures and Lisfranc injuries, as well as osteochondral lesions and arthritis [10].

Magnetic Resonance Imaging (MRI). This modality is particularly useful in the assessment of soft tissues, ligaments, and tendons. In the foot and ankle, MRI is particularly useful for evaluation the ligaments around the ankle such as the deltoid ligament, ATFL, and PTFL in cases of ankle instability [9].

8.4   Other Investigations

Nerve Conduction Test. A nerve conduction test is useful for evaluating suspected nerve entrapment [10].

8.4.1   Algorithm for Lower Leg, Foot, and Ankle Assessment

This algorithm (Fig. 8.23) is a mind map for simplifying the approach of lower leg, foot, and ankle problems according to patient complain and virtual assessment of elbow and forearm.

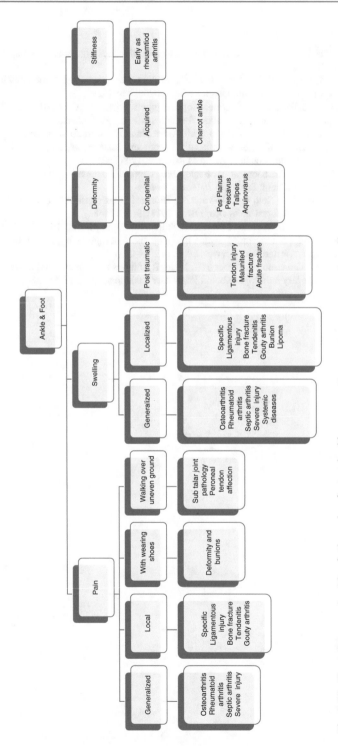

Fig. 8.23 Chart shows an algorithm for lower leg, foot, and ankle assessment

References

1. Dawe EJ, Davis J. Anatomy and biomechanics of the foot and ankle. Orthop Trauma. 2011;25(4):279–86.
2. Chang AL, Mandell JC. Syndesmotic ligaments of the ankle: anatomy, multimodality imaging, and patterns of injury. Curr Probl Diagn Radiol. 2020;49(6):452–9.
3. Trnka HJ, Lara JS. Freiberg's infraction: surgical options. Foot Ankle Clin. 2019;24(4):669–76.
4. Amendola A. Physical examination of the foot and ankle. In: Musculoskeletal physical examination E-Book: an evidence-based approach. Amsterdam: Elsevier; 2016. p. 199.
5. Alazzawi S, Sukeik M, King D, Vemulapalli K. Foot and ankle history and clinical examination: a guide to everyday practice. World J Orthop. 2017;8(1):21.
6. Lampley AJ, Gross CE, Klement M, Easley ME. Clinical examination. In: Foot and ankle sports orthopaedics. Cham: Springer; 2016. p. 39–48.
7. Pinto JA, Saito E, Lira Neto OA, Rowinski S, Blumetti FC, Dobashi ET. Foot print study in children during the Jack test. Acta Ortop Bras. 2011;19(3):125–8.
8. Thompson TC. A test for rupture of the tendo achillis. Acta Orthop Scand. 1962;32(1–4):461–5.
9. Deakins-Roche M, Fredericson M, Kraus E. Ankle and foot injuries in runners. In: Clinical care of the runner. Amsterdam: Elsevier; 2020. p. 231–45.
10. Thierfelder KM, Gemescu IN, Weber MA, Meier R. Injuries of ligaments and tendons of foot and ankle: what every radiologist should know. Der Radiologe. 2018;58(5):415–21.

Spine

9

Khaled M. Emara, Shady Abdelghaffar Mahmoud,
Kevin Zhai, and Thomas Mroz

9.1   History Taking

History is a vital step that can provide clues to reach the definitive diagnosis via telemedicine.

9.2   Personal History

Age of the patient and the onset of complaints can provide clue to the diagnosis. Deformity of progressive course in adolescence can suggest scoliosis while obese old age with back pain radiating to the extremity can suggest spondylosis [1].

Certain **occupation and sport activities** are at higher risk for spinal disorders. History of heavy lifting can predispose to intervertebral disc herniation. Young gymnastics are at risk for spondylolisthesis [2].

K. M. Emara
Department of Orthopedic Surgery, Ain Shams University, Cairo, Egypt

S. A. Mahmoud (✉)
Orthopedic Surgery, Ain Shams University, Cairo, Egypt

K. Zhai · T. Mroz
Department of Orthopedic Surgery, Cleveland Clinic Foundation, Cleveland, OH, USA

© The Author(s), under exclusive license to Springer Nature Switzerland AG 2022   109
K. M. Emara, N. S. Piuzzi (eds.), *The Principles of Virtual Orthopedic Assessment*,
https://doi.org/10.1007/978-3-030-80402-2_9

9.3   Present History

9.3.1   Pain

Low back pain alone affects up to 80% of the population at some point in life, and 1–2% of the United States adult population is disabled because of such pain [3, 4]. It can be for simplicity classified into three main categories:

1. Result from local spine disorder like infection, tumor, deformity, and mechanical.
2. Associated with nerve root irritation and/or compression as intervertebral disc.
3. Back and leg pain of lumbar canal stenosis.

Analysis of pain can help to put the case preliminary into the appropriate category and hence reach the diagnosis.

- **Onset, course, and duration**: sudden onset is more suggestive to mechanical factors.
- **Site, radiation, and character**: dull aching pain, heaviness in the spine or para spinal region may indicate muscle sprain or mechanical pain. Mechanical pain can radiate to the buttocks and back of thigh but not extend below the knee. Contrarily, sharp knife-like pain from the back and shooting, usually, to one side lower limb especially below the knee (in L4, 5, S1 nerve roots irritation) usually signify the presence of nerve irritation due to disc prolapse or spondylosis.
- **Intensity**: Quantify the intensity of the pain on a numerical scale from 1 to 10 can provide an idea about significance of pain. Severe pain may result from nerve root irritation, tumor, or infection process. Mild pain especially after twisting incident may indicate muscle sprain.
- **Impact**: another measure for the severity is the effect of this pain on the daily routine, work, and sleep.
- **What aggravates and what relieves**: Pain that increases with activities, twisting, and bending are usually of mechanical origin. This pain commonly relieved with resting and at night. In contrast to pain due to tumor or infection origin that may be constant and nocturnal [4, 5].

Pain that increases with leaning forward or straining increases the suspicion of disc prolapse, while that relieved with sitting suggest spinal canal stenosis [6, 7].

Numbness: distribution, onset, course, and duration are important to localize the affected nerve roots.

Weakness: in the form of difficult ambulation or inadequate upper or lower limb function. Lower limb weakness with decreased hand dexterity can suggest myelopathy. Significant weakness of nerve root distribution signifies the degree of compression and may indicate the need of surgical intervention.

Bowel/Bladder symptoms and sexual symptoms: Is mandatory to be asked to exclude possible development of cauda equina, one of the rare emergencies in spine (incidence is between 1 in 33,000 and 1 in 100,000) that mandates emergent intervention.

Deformity (kyphoscoliosis) and **limping** (e.g., because of pelvic tilt).

Stiffness: especially in the morning may associate inflammatory etiology as rheumatoid arthritis and ankylosing spondylitis.

Affection of other joints: Associated rheumatoid hand may suggest rheumatoid arthritis etiology for the cervical condition.

9.3.2   History of Trauma

Walking distance: decreased walking distance suggests lumbar canal stenosis.

Constitutional symptoms: fever, nocturnal sweating, pain, and cachexia may indicate infection etiology as tuberculosis.

9.4   Past History

9.4.1   Medications

Surgical history: provide insight regarding the previous scars and the possible difficulties that are anticipated in the future surgeries if needed.

Medical history: History of certain diseases as rheumatoid arthritis, tuberculosis is important to outline the possible diagnosis. Psychosocial factors and emotional distress should also be assessed, as they are strong predictors of poor outcomes.

9.5   Clinical Examination

9.5.1   Inspection

Exposure by undressing to underwear as possible is required to inspect the whole spine (Fig. 9.1).

Inspect for skin **scars**, **sinuses**, **discoloration**, and **swellings** (Figs. 9.2, 9.3, and 9.4).

Deformity should be inspected in the sagittal (Fig. 9.5) and coronal view (Figs. 9.1 and 9.6):

Normal sagittal curvature are cervical lordosis (20–40°), thoracic kyphosis (20–50°), and lumbar lordosis (averages 60°). Cervicothoracic kyphosis is suggestive of ankylosing spondylitis, increased thoracic kyphosis is suggestive for osteoporotic fractures in elderly and Scheuermann disease in young age. While lost

Fig. 9.1 Patient's exposure for spine assessment. Deformity assessment from front coronal view can be also inspected

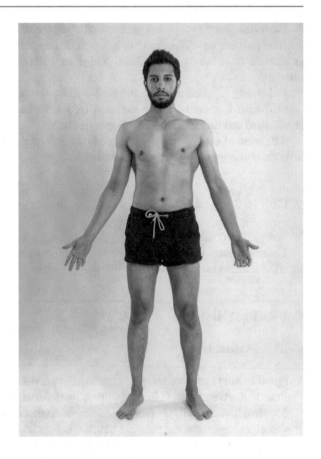

lumbar lordosis may represent a protective spasm to the underlying degenerative disease or posterior pelvic tilt as in case of tight hamstrings, exaggerated lumbar lordosis may suggest spondylolisthesis or compensatory to anterior pelvic tilt with short iliopsoas or compensatory to thoracic kyphosis (Fig. 9.5) [4].

Coronal alignment assessment should be in systematic descending manner looking for head position, hair line, neck position, shoulders, scapulae level, torso-arm angle, spine furrow line, pelvis, and glutei (Figs. 9.1 and 9.6). This assessment can be facilitated by a software that outlines the plumb line to detect any deviation. If in query, forward bending test is done to reveal rib hump, if present, more clearly indicating scoliosis.

Tuft of hair should also be searched for that may accompany neurofibromatosis or meningocele cases.

Gait should follow the inspection: The type of gait can provide clue for the diagnosis. For example, short step gait can indicate back muscle spasm, unsteady gait for myelopathy, and sciatica gait (with extended hips and flexed knee) for nerve root tension as lumbar disc prolapse [3, 4].

Fig. 9.2 Inspect for skin lesions from the front

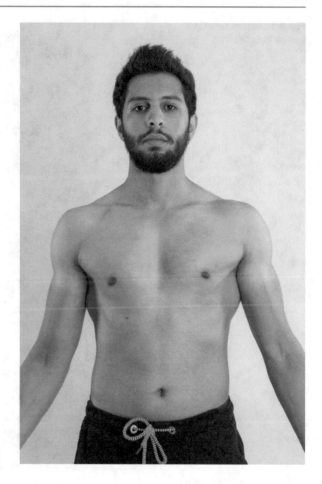

Walking on heels (Fig. 9.7) and toes (Fig. 9.8) are beneficial to assess the motor power roughly of L4 and S1 nerve roots, respectively.

9.5.2 Palpation

It cannot be assessed by telemedicine. However, the patient is instructed to draw the possible sites of pain using black marker. This may be of help to determine the tender points as a substitute to the palpation. Another method is to provide the patient with a drawing chart containing the required site of compression helped by a caregiver to elicit tenderness (Fig. 9.9) [4].

Fig. 9.3 Inspect for skin
lesions from the back

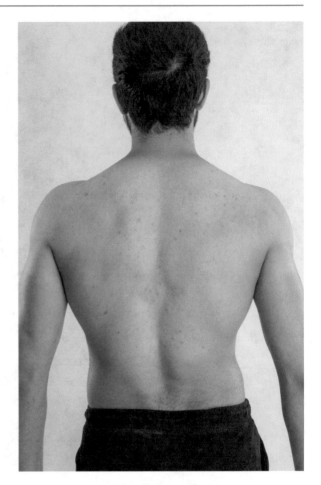

9.5.3   Range of Motion

The use of well-designed software in telemedicine can accurately assess the range
of motion and save the data precisely for follow-up comparison and research
conduct.

9.5.4   Cervical

With the camera looking to the sagittal view of neck:

Flexion: Ask the patient to put chin to chest. Measure the distance between them
using a virtual ruler (Fig. 9.10).

Extension: Ask the patient to look to the ceiling. Normally the face can be parallel to the ceiling. If not measure the angle between the face and the horizontal line
using goniometer-based software (Fig. 9.11).

Fig. 9.4 Inspect for skin lesions from the side

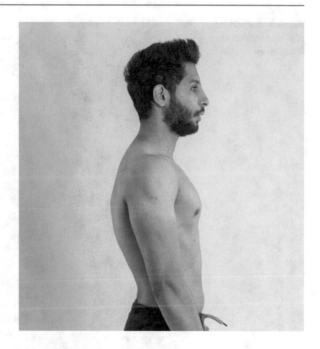

With the camera looking to the coronal view of neck:

Lateral bending: Ask the patient to touch ear to shoulder. Measure the distance between them using a virtual ruler (Fig. 9.12).

Rotation: Ask the patient to rotate chin to shoulder.

9.5.5 Thoracolumbar

Flexion: ask the patient to lean forward with extended knees. Measure the flexion degree by finger to floor distance or angle formed between the back and a vertical line utilizing the suitable software. Limited painful flexion may indicate disc prolapse (Fig. 9.13) [3, 4].

Extension: ask the patient to extend the back as possible. Again, measure the extension degree by an angle between the back and a vertical line. Limited painful extension may indicate lumbar canal stenosis (Fig. 9.14) [4].

Lateral bending: ask the patient to lean laterally and advance the fingers down the legs with extended knees. The degree of bending measured by finger to floor distance or an angle between the trunk and a vertical line (Fig. 9.15) [4].

Rotation: thoracic rotation can be assessed with sited patient and putting the camera at a higher level. So, looking from the top view. The degree of rotation is measured by angle between shoulder plane and the coronal plane (Fig. 9.16) [3].

Fig. 9.5 Inspect for
sagittal plane spine
deformities

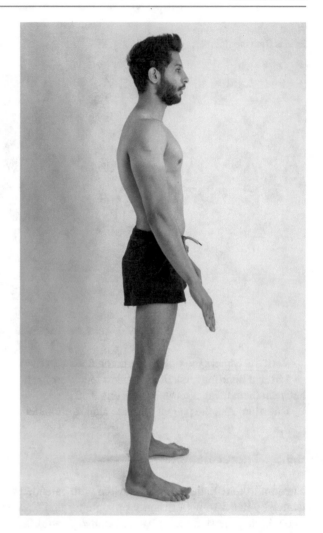

9.6   Neurological Assessment

9.6.1   Sensory Assessment

It is difficult to assess the sensory disturbance distribution and reflexes via telemedicine. However, a chart of upper and lower limbs localizing the dermatomes at clear easily located points to be assessed by a caregiver using cotton while comparing both sides with the patient closed eye. This provide a clue regarding the possible level of nerve root affection (Figs. 9.17, 9.18, 9.19, and 9.20) [8].

We will depend on history of numbness and its accurate location to provide a clue as regard the level of affected nerve roots.

Fig. 9.6 Inspect for
coronal plane spine
deformities

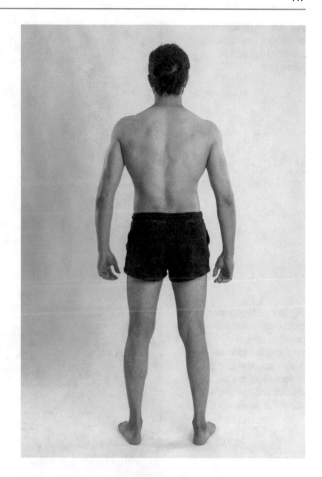

Fig. 9.7 Walking on heels
provides a clue on the
motor power of L4
nerve root

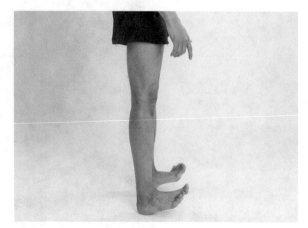

Fig. 9.8 Walking on toes provides a clue on the motor power of S1 nerve root

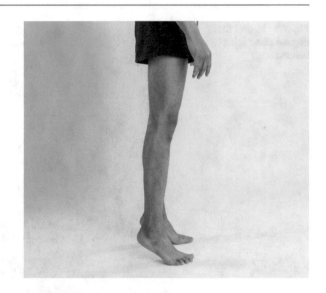

Fig. 9.9 Diagrammatic chart demonstrates the possible sites of compression to locate pain. 1: spinous process region, 2: paraspinal region, 3: sacrum and coccyx, 4: sacroiliac joints

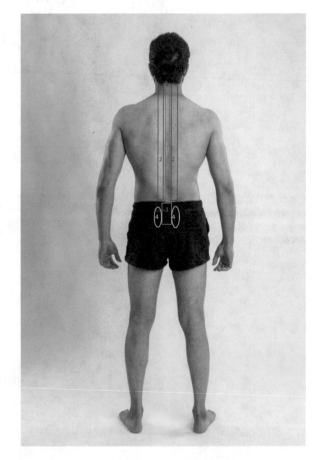

Fig. 9.10 Cervical flexion range

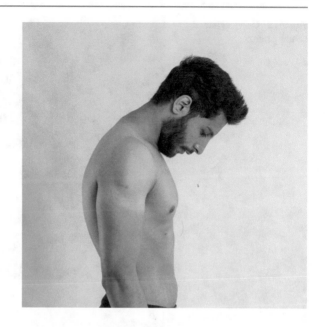

Fig. 9.11 Cervical extension range

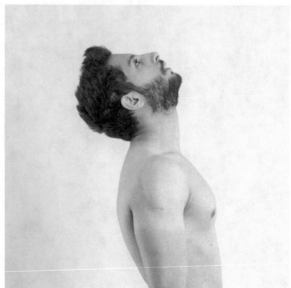

Fig. 9.12 Cervical lateral
bending range

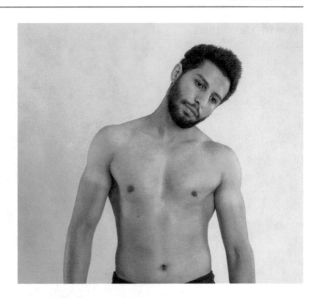

Fig. 9.13 Thoracolumbar
flexion range

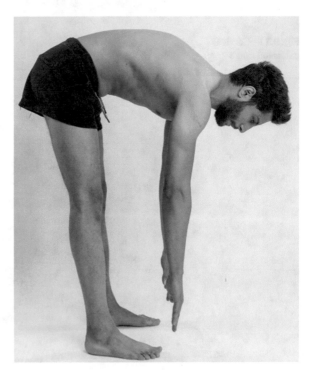

Fig. 9.14 Thoracolumbar extension range

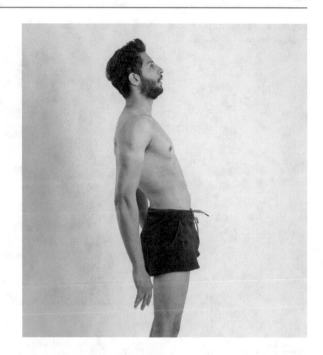

Fig. 9.15 Thoracolumbar lateral bending range

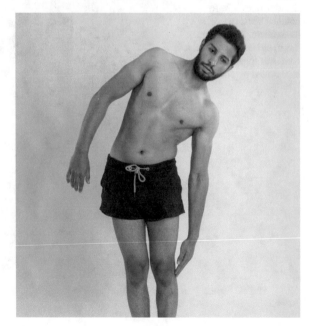

Fig. 9.16 Thoracic
rotation range

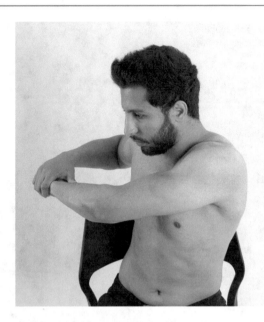

Fig. 9.17 Photo
demonstrates how to
conduct sensory
assessment. The patient
has to close his eyes and a
caregiver touch the area of
assessment by cotton

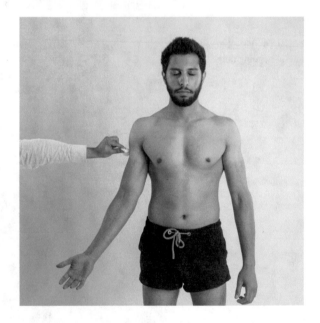

Fig. 9.18 Upper limb chart demonstrates the dermatomes. 1: C5 sensory dermatome, 2: C6 sensory dermatome, 3: C7 sensory dermatome, 4: C8 sensory dermatome, 5: T1 sensory dermatome, 6: T2 sensory dermatome

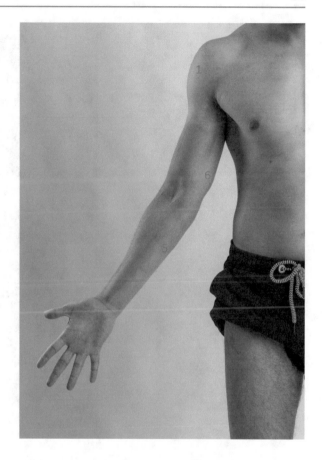

9.6.2 Motor Assessment

It can be estimated by using simple measures to exclude weakness:

9.6.3 Cervical

It is difficult to be assessed using telemedicine as the caregiver will feel the resistance not the physician, but motor power estimation can be determined roughly. If the patient can do the movement against resistance, then his muscle grading is three or more. If any degree of resistance offered, the grade will be four or more.

C5: Ask the patient to flex the elbow while a caregiver tries to resist it (Fig. 9.21).

C7: Ask the patient to extend the elbow while a caregiver tries to resist it (Fig. 9.22).

Fig. 9.19 Lower limb chart demonstrates the dermatomes front view. 1: L1 sensory dermatome, 2: L2 sensory dermatome, 3: L3 sensory dermatome, 4: L4 sensory dermatome, 5: L5 sensory dermatome, 6: S1 sensory dermatome

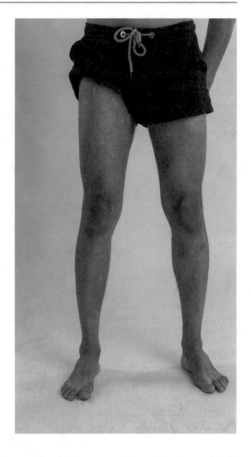

C6: Ask the patient to extend the wrist while a caregiver tries to resist it (Fig. 9.23).

C8: Ask the patient to flex the fingers while a caregiver tries to resist it (Fig. 9.24).

T1: Ask the patient to abduct the fingers while a caregiver tries to resist it (Fig. 9.25).

9.6.4 Lumbar

L1,2: Ask the patient to sit then elevating the hip maximally while a caregiver tries to resist it (Fig. 9.26).

L3: Ask the patient to lie supine with flexed knee on a hard triangle making the knee flexed 30 then ask the patient to extend it completely (Fig. 9.27).

L4: walk on heels (Fig. 9.7).

L5: lie on the side and ask to elevate the limb with extended knees. A caregiver can try to resist it (Fig. 9.28).

S1: walk on tip toes (Fig. 9.8) [8].

Fig. 9.20 Lower limb chart demonstrates the dermatomes back view. 1,2: S2 sensory dermatome, 3: S3 sensory dermatome, 4: S4 sensory dermatome

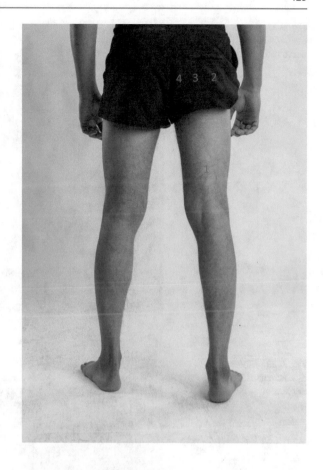

Fig. 9.21 Motor assessment of C5 nerve root

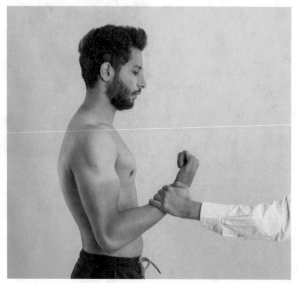

Fig. 9.22 Motor
assessment of C7
nerve root

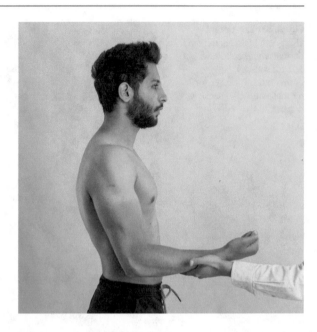

Fig. 9.23 Motor
assessment of C6
nerve root

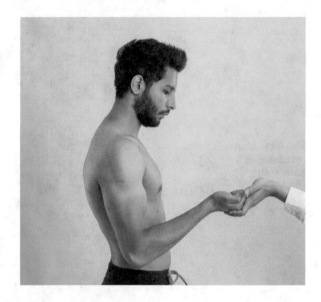

Fig. 9.24 Motor assessment of C8 nerve root

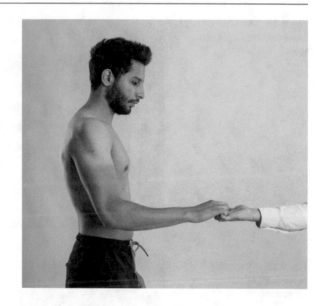

Fig. 9.25 Motor assessment of T1 nerve root

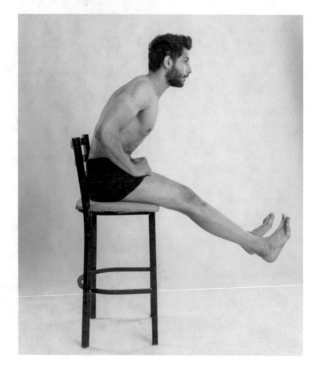

Fig. 9.26 Motor
assessment of L1,2 nerve
roots

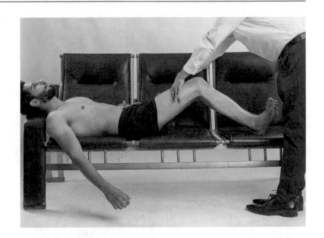

Fig. 9.27 Motor
assessment of L3
nerve root

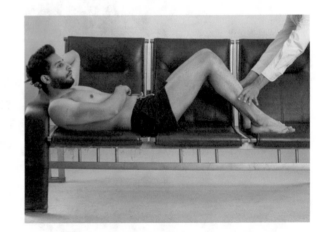

Fig. 9.28 Motor
assessment of L5
nerve root

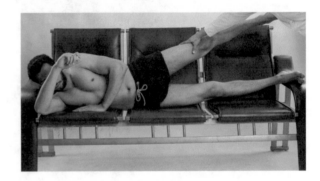

9.7 Special Tests

9.7.1 Shoulder Abduction Test

It is very important test to differentiate shoulder pain from cervical radiculopathy pain. Improvement of the pain upon shoulder abduction suggests cervical radiculopathy [9].

9.7.2 Lhermitte Test

It is helpful to diagnose cervical myelopathy. Ask the caregiver to flex the neck of the patient passively. Shock-line sensation radiating down the spinal axis to arms and/or legs (Fig. 9.29) [10].

Fig. 9.29 Lhermitte test

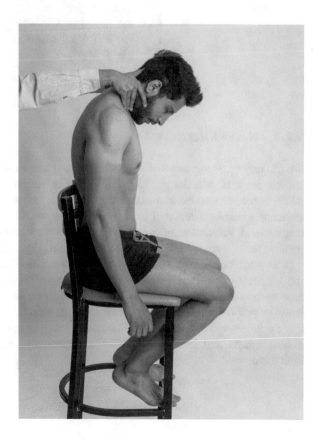

Fig. 9.30 Slump test

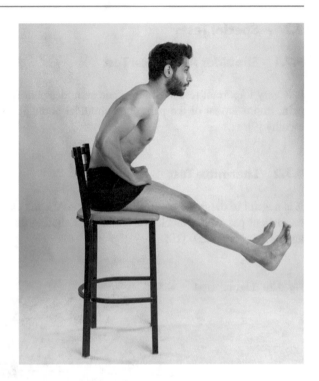

9.7.3   Nerve Stretch Test

We can rely on Slump test to diagnose nerve root stretch via telemedicine instead of straight leg test. Ask the patient to sit on the couch edge, lean the trunk forward while the neck extended to maintain forward gaze, extend the knee actively as possible and ask for existence of pain and if present where is it exactly to confirm the diagnosis. A Valsalva maneuver while the knee is extended may be asked that can confirm nerve stretch by exaggeration of the pain (Fig. 9.30) [9].

It is worth noting that we will depend on the judicious use of imaging to confirm the suspected diagnosis made with telemedicine. Nevertheless, we recommend face-to-face assessment whenever you are still in doubt especially in complicated cases or before surgical intervention. However, with telemedicine assessment, we can exclude serious disorders and diagnose many common benign disorders like muscle spasm and intervertebral disc and prescribe medications effectively to treat them.

9.8   Investigation

Depending on data of history and virtual physical examination. These may include:

9.8.1   Imaging

Imaging will be used judiciously to confirm the diagnosis in telemedicine. These may include:

Spinal X-rays to look for spinal fractures, disk problems, infections, tumors, and bone spurs.

Magnetic resonance imaging (MRI) or **computed tomography (CT) scans** are used to see detailed images of bone and soft tissues of the back. An MRI can show pressure on a nerve, disk herniation, and any arthritic condition that might be pressing on a nerve. MRIs are usually ordered to confirm the diagnosis of sciatica.

Nerve conduction velocity studies/electromyography examine how well electrical impulses travel through the sciatic nerve and the response of muscles.

Myelogram to determine if a vertebrae or disk is causing the pain [3, 4].

9.8.2   Laboratory

CBC, ESR, CRP in suspected infection.

9.8.3   Algorithm for Low Back Pain Assessment

A mind map can be followed to reach the diagnosis. For simplicity, pain can be localized to the back, associated with leg pain of radiculopathy, or associated with leg pain and claudication of spinal canal stenosis. Psychologic pain is the diagnosis of exclusion.

References

1. Huston CW, McCowen SA. Etiologies of painful spinal disorders. In: DePalma MJ, editor. Spine evidence based interventional spine. 1st ed. New York: Demos Medical Publishing; 2011. p. 10.
2. Rudwaleit M, van der Heijde D, Landewé R, et al. The development of assessment of spondyloarthritis international society classification criteria for axial spondyloarthritis (parts I & II). Ann Rheum Dis. 2009;68:770–83.
3. Barr KP, Harast MA. Low back pain. In: Braddom RL, editor. Physical medicine and rehabilitation. 4th ed. Philadelphia: Elsevier Saunders; 2011. p. 871.
4. Chou R, Qaseem A, Snow V, et al. Diagnosis and treatment of low back pain: a joint clinical practice guideline from the American College of Physicians and the American Pain Society. Ann Intern Med. 2007;147:478–91.
5. Deyo RA, Weinstein JN. Low back pain. N Engl J Med. 2001;344(5):363–70.
6. Lurie J, Tomkins-Lane C. Management of lumbar spinal stenosis. BMJ. 2016;352:h6234.
7. Whitman J, Flynn T, Fritz J. Nonsurgical management of patients with lumbar spinal stenosis: a literature review and a case series of three patients managed with physical therapy. Phys Med Rehabil Clin N Am. 2003;14(1):77–101, vi–vii.
8. Thoomes EJ, van Geest S, van der Windt DA, et al. Value of physical tests in diagnosing cervical radiculopathy: a systematic review. Spine J. 2018;18(1):179–89.
9. Fast A, Parikh S, Marin EL. The shoulder abduction relief sign in cervical radiculopathy. Arch Phys Med Rehabil. 1989;70:402–3.
10. Schmalstieg WF, Weinshenker BG. Approach to acute or subacute myelopathy. Neurol Clin Pract. 2010;75(Suppl 1):S2–8.

Dealing with Children and Noncompliant Patients

10

Mohamed Noureldeen Essa, Kevin Zhai, and Dominic King

10.1 History

Telemedicine appointments can provide an opportunity not only to ask questions and obtain a full history, but also to reassure parents and address any anxiety they may have regarding normal variations of their child's development. It is important for the surgeon to establish rapport and build a bond with the child during the visit, using resources like cartoons to help child engagement [2].

Age. The age of the child is crucial for developing a differential diagnosis. Hip symptoms in a 7-year-old boy with delayed bone age can suggest Perthes disease, whereas hip symptoms in an obese 13-year-old boy should raise suspicion for a slipped capital femoral epiphysis (SCFE) [3, 4].

Birth Order. Developmental dysplasia of the hip (DDH) and familial diseases can be affected by birth order [5].

Birth History. Birth history is an important consideration especially when neuromuscular conditions such as cerebral palsy are suspected. Birth history can be divided into the prenatal, natal, and postnatal periods. In the prenatal period, any history of maternal infection in the first trimester or vaginal bleeding may provide a clue for possible brain injury that could lead to cerebral palsy. Medications in the first trimester and diabetes can also be associated with birth abnormalities. Decreased fetal kicks in late pregnancy can be associated with arthrogryposis. Important factors to consider for the natal period include the birth weight, type of presentation, mode of delivery, site of delivery (home or hospital), any birth injuries, and whether the child was delivered full-term or pre-term. Postnatally, any neonatal jaundice

M. N. Essa (✉)
Al Bank Al-Ahly Hospital, Cairo, Egypt

K. Zhai · D. King
Department of Orthopedic Surgery, Cleveland Clinic Foundation, Cleveland, OH, USA

© The Author(s), under exclusive license to Springer Nature Switzerland AG 2022
K. M. Emara, N. S. Piuzzi (eds.), *The Principles of Virtual Orthopedic Assessment*,
https://doi.org/10.1007/978-3-030-80402-2_10

necessitating UV light intervention, need for neonatal ICU, incidence of hypoxia or cyanosis, and APGAR score should be noted [6].

Past History. It is important to consider a broad history in the pediatric patient. A medical history of systemic diseases like renal disease with associated renal osteodystrophy, immunization status, and previous hospitalizations may all play an important role in establishing a diagnosis. Surgical history may provide insight regarding previous scars and help the surgeon anticipate any possible difficulties for future surgeries. Family history can be an important way to detect diseases such as neurofibromatosis, Charcot–Marie–Tooth disease, Friedreich ataxia, and dysplasia. A nutritional history is important to consider as well, especially in the pediatric patient, and may help identify nutritional rickets as the underlying etiology for deformities in toddlers. Finally, developmental history with both physical and mental milestones can be useful to obtain, particularly in suspected cases of neurodevelopmental disorders [7].

Pain. An analysis of pain, though less helpful for younger children who are not verbal, can be useful for older children and adolescents. Any sudden onset of pain is typically suggestive of mechanical etiologies. The intensity of pain as quantified on a numerical 1–10 scale and its impact on daily routines like school and sleep can both give an indication of pain significance. Pain that is aggravated by activities and relieved by rest can suggest arthritis. Pain that is due to a neoplastic or infectious etiology is more commonly constant in nature and can be nocturnal. The specific site of pain and any radiation of the pain may be of diagnostic utility as well [8].

Gait. Any limping gait may be indicative of pain, and can be caused by infection, trauma, or unstable SCFE. The age of onset and the course of limping can help to narrow the differential diagnosis. Limping during walking age may suggest developmental dysplasia of the hip, for example. Any constitutional symptoms are suggestive of systemic infection, and a history of respiratory tract infection can be suggestive of transient synovitis. Other abnormal gaits like out-toeing may indicate SCFE, while in-toeing may suggest excessive femoral anteversion, tibial in-torsion, or metatarsus adductus [9, 10].

Deformity. The site, age of onset, character, and any associated pain with any deformities should be determined. For example, a painless flexible flat foot deformity in childhood is usually idiopathic while painful rigid flat foot in adolescence may suggest tarsal coalition. Coronal knee deformities may be part of normal development or they may be pathological as in nutritional rickets or Blount's disease. As a general rule, any rapidly progressive or asymmetrical deformity should prompt a search for underlying pathology [7, 8].

Other. Other symptoms like swelling, stiffness, and weakness should be assessed as well. The presence of any constitutional symptoms like fever, chills, or fatigue may suggest an infectious etiology. Finally, it is important to inquire about any history of traumatic physical injuries that may be the cause of angulated deformities or limb length discrepancies [7, 8].

10.2   Examination

Virtual clinical assessment should include a general examination to detect any syndromes that may affect multiple regions of the body, as well as a focused assessment on the affected limb. The child should be undressed to underwear to investigate a lower limb disorder, and the shirt should be removed in the case of an upper limb disorder.

General Examination. Observe for any abnormal facies as may occur in Down syndrome, blue sclera that can suggest osteogenesis imperfecta, and abnormalities in height or proportions that can suggest dysplasia. Other general findings to look for include café au lait spots and axillary freckling that are characteristic of neurofibromatosis, tufts of hair at the back which may indicate meningomyelocele, and vascular markings that may suggest Klippel Trenaunay syndrome. Any kyphoscoliosis should be observed and noted as well [8].

Inspection. Observe the child anteriorly, posteriorly, and laterally. Observe for any skin swellings, scars, sinuses, wasting, and discoloration. Next, using a straight plumb line, observe joint alignment to determine whether the patient has a symmetrical shoulder level, symmetrical scapulae, and a level pelvis. Search for any possible coronal knee deformities, and document intermalleolar and intercondylar distance. Observe for other potential knee deformities including squinting patellae due to excessive femoral anteversion, ankle deformities, and deformities of the forefoot, midfoot, and hindfoot. A similar systematic sequence can be applied to the upper limb in searching for any skin or muscle abnormalities, deformities, or abnormal postures [8].

Gait. If the child is walking, gait analysis can be performed. To do so, inspect gait from the coronal and sagittal views while observing the appearance of the hip, knee, and foot. This can be especially important in the setting of neuromuscular diseases to interpret any findings of spastic or shortened muscle units. At the level of the hip, search for any possible anterior or posterior pelvic tilt, scissoring of the thighs, or a tilted pelvis. At the knee level, look for any coronal knee deformities, squinting patellae, and any flexed knee gait. At the foot and ankle level, look for equines, pes planovalgus or pes cavovarus, forefoot abduction, big toe deformities, and coronal ankle deformities. Observe for general patterns of gait deformities as well, as these may be indicative of neuromuscular diseases: jumping gait, crouch gait, equines gait, ataxic gait, and circumduction gaits. Other abnormal gaits that may be encountered in pediatric populations include antalgic gait that may occur in a painful condition, Trendelenburg gait that may occur in the setting of hip diseases like DDH or coxa vara, short limb gait in a limb length discrepancy, out-toeing gait which may be seen in SCFE, and high steppage gait that often occurs in knee flexion deformities [4, 5, 10].

Palpation. Palpation cannot be assessed directly by telemedicine. However, the patient and their guardian can identify possible sites of pain and mark these with a black marker. This can be used as a proxy for determining sites of tenderness. Alternatively, the parents can be provided with an anatomical chart with required sites of compression to elicit tenderness, and this can be performed during the telemedicine visit.

Range of Motion. Active ROM can be assessed in older children and adolescents. (See previous chapters for how to perform active ROM assessment for each joint.) Passive ROM can be assessed virtually by asking the caregiver to manipulate each joint in front of the camera.

Limb Length Measurements. The Galeazzi test can be effectively translated to telemedicine. Ask the patient to lie supine and then flex both knees and hips to 45°. A static image can be taken from the top and the side views, which can then be used to interpret the cause of limb length discrepancy.

Another way to know limb length discrepancy is that in the normal patient the heels should be levelled, and the plane of the anterior superior iliac spines at right angles to the edge of the couch. Where there is significant true shortening the heels will not be levelled (the discrepancy is a guide to the amount of shortening) and pelvis will not be tilted. The site and amount of shortening must now be further investigated [10].

However, as the degree of limb length discrepancy cannot be directly measured, a CT scanogram is recommended to accurately determine the degree and the site of shortening.

Neuromuscular Assessment. Start the assessment by inspecting the patient while standing and observing their gait if ambulatory. If the patient is not ambulatory, begin the examination with the patient in the sitting or supine position. From these positions, search for any involuntary movements such as dyskinesia, athetosis, and ataxia. Gross motor functional classification system (GMFCS) can also be assessed [6].

To differentiate between increased tone and contracture, the caregiver can be asked to move the examined joint once slowly, once rapidly, and then repeatedly 3–5 times. A provisional estimation of the affected muscles and bones can be made virtually although it is very difficult to assess the muscle power, tone, and contracture accurately in a virtual setting. Thus, it is almost inevitable that these patients will need face-to-face assessment especially prior to commencing physiotherapy programs, orthosis, or surgical intervention.

10.3 Radiology

Plain Film X-Ray (PXR). PXR of the affected region can be obtained in the AP, oblique, and lateral views to look for fractures, arthritis, congenital deformities, instability, and infections. Scanograms can be used to measure limb length discrepancy and to the site and degree of discrepancy [11].

Computed Tomography (CT). CT scans can provide detailed images of the bone which may be useful in conditions like tarsal coalition. CT scanograms can also measure limb length discrepancy even in the presence of deformities. The CT modality is also useful in measuring the rotational profile of the extremities [11].

Magnetic Resonance Imaging (MRI). MRI allows for detailed assessment of the soft tissue, including tendons and ligaments. It is especially useful in assessing avascular necrosis.

Ultrasound. Ultrasound is useful for detecting joint effusions in suspected infections and to assess tendinous and ligamentous lesions.

10.4 Other Investigations

Nerve Conduction Test and **Electromyogram.** Both of these can be useful in the diagnosis of nerve injuries as well as follow-up analysis for nerve regeneration.

Gait Lab. This can be especially useful in neuromuscular cases.

Laboratory Studies. CBC, ESR, and CRP can be useful in detecting the presence of infection. A metabolic profile and Vitamin D can be useful in the evaluation of nutritional rickets and SCFE. Renal function tests should be ordered if renal osteodystrophy is suspected. Finally, a serum CK-MB test should be ordered if muscle dystrophy is suspected.

10.5 Algorithm

Given the heterogeneous set of potential abnormalities that present in a pediatric assessment, the following algorithm can be used to accelerate the evaluation and diagnostic process (Fig. 10.1).

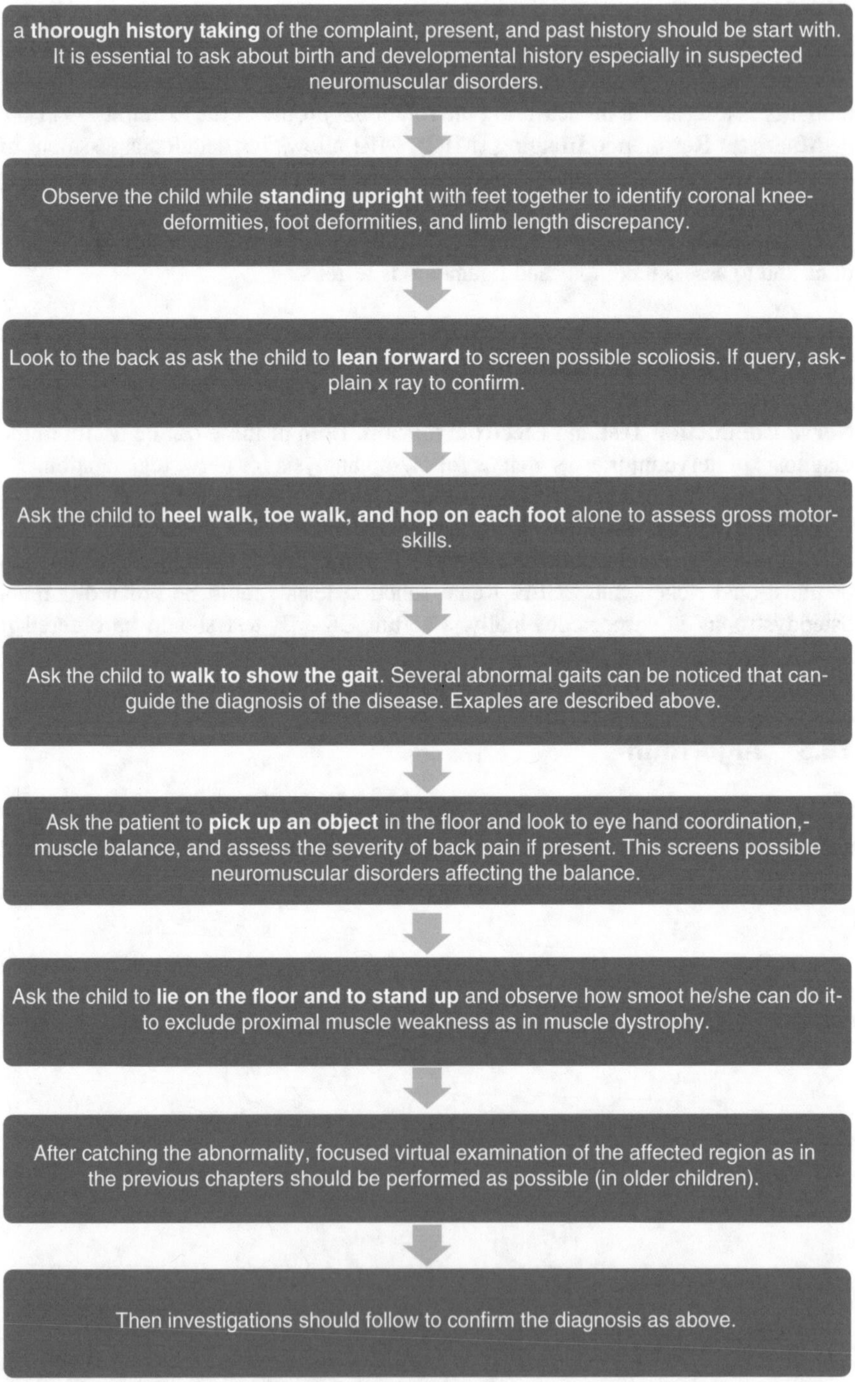

a **thorough history taking** of the complaint, present, and past history should be start with. It is essential to ask about birth and developmental history especially in suspected neuromuscular disorders.

Observe the child while **standing upright** with feet together to identify coronal knee-deformities, foot deformities, and limb length discrepancy.

Look to the back as ask the child to **lean forward** to screen possible scoliosis. If query, ask-plain x ray to confirm.

Ask the child to **heel walk, toe walk, and hop on each foot** alone to assess gross motor-skills.

Ask the child to **walk to show the gait**. Several abnormal gaits can be noticed that can-guide the diagnosis of the disease. Exaples are described above.

Ask the patient to **pick up an object** in the floor and look to eye hand coordination,-muscle balance, and assess the severity of back pain if present. This screens possible neuromuscular disorders affecting the balance.

Ask the child to **lie on the floor and to stand up** and observe how smoot he/she can do it-to exclude proximal muscle weakness as in muscle dystrophy.

After catching the abnormality, focused virtual examination of the affected region as in the previous chapters should be performed as possible (in older children).

Then investigations should follow to confirm the diagnosis as above.

Fig. 10.1 Chart demonstrates how to conduct teleassessment of pediatrics

References

1. Daruwalla ZJ, Wong KL, Thambiah J. The application of telemedicine in orthopedic surgery in Singapore: a pilot study on a secure, mobile telehealth application and messaging platform. JMIR Mhealth Uhealth. 2014;2(2):e28.
2. Gordon JE, Schoenecker PL, Osland JD, et al. Smoking and socio-economic status in the etiology and severity of Legg-Calvé- Perthes' disease. J Pediatr Orthop B. 2004;13:367.
3. Peck D, Voss LM, Voss TT. Slipped capital femoral epiphysis: diagnosis and management. Am Fam Physician. 2017;95(12):779–84.
4. American Academy of Pediatrics. Clinical practice guideline: early detection of developmental dysplasia of the hip. Committee on Quality Improvement, Subcommittee on Developmental Dysplasia of the Hip. Pediatrics. 2000;105:896.
5. Pearl PL, Sable C, Evans S, et al. International telemedicine consultations for neurodevelopmental disabilities. Telemed e-Health. 2014;20(6):559–62.
6. Camasta CA, Graeser TA. Tarsal coalition and pes planovalgus: clinical examination, diagnostic imaging, and surgical planning. In: The pediatric foot and ankle. Cham: Springer; 2020. p. 191–218.
7. Sarup S. Common orthopedic problems in children. In: Pediatric rheumatology. Berlin: Springer; 2017. p. 181–99.
8. Kahf H, Kesbeh Y, van Baarsel E, Patel V, Alonzo N. Approach to pediatric rotational limb deformities. Orthop Rev. 2019;11(3):8118.
9. Terry MA, Winell JJ, Green DW, et al. Measurement variance in limb length discrepancy: clinical and radiographic assessment of interobserver and intraobserver variability. J Pediatr Orthop. 2005;25(2):197–201.
10. Medina LS, Applegate KE, Blackmore CC, editors. Evidence-based imaging in pediatrics: optimizing imaging in pediatric patient care. Cham: Springer; 2010.
11. Cohen MD. Clinical utility of magnetic resonance imaging in pediatrics. Am J Dis Child. 1986;140(9):947–56.

Correction to: The Principles of Virtual Orthopedic Assessment

Khaled M. Emara and Nicolas S. Piuzzi

Correction to:
K. M. Emara, N. S. Piuzzi (eds.), ***The***
Principles of Virtual Orthopedic Assessment,
https://doi.org/10.1007/978-3-030-80402-2

The author Keith Diamond was incorrectly included in the author group of Chapter 3 "Shoulder and Upper Arm" instead of Chapter 4 "Elbow and Forearm" in the initially published version. The author group has been corrected now in both the chapters.

The updated original versions of the chapters can be found at
https://doi.org/10.1007/978-3-030-80402-2_3
https://doi.org/10.1007/978-3-030-80402-2_4

Printed in the United States
by Baker & Taylor Publisher Services